T0221252

RELIGION AND THE CURE OF SOULS IN JUNG'S PSYCHOLOGY

Founded by C. K. Ogden

The International Library of Psychology

ANALYTICAL PSYCHOLOGY
In 12 Volumes

RELIGION AND THE CURE OF SOULS IN JUNG'S PSYCHOLOGY

HANS SCHAER

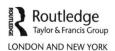

Routledge
Taylor & Francis Group

LONDON AND NEW YORK

First published in 1951
by Routledge

Reprinted in 1999
by Routledge
2 Park Square, Milton Park, Abingdon, Oxfordshire OX14 4RN
711 Third Avenue, New York, NY 10017
Transferred to Digital Printing 2007
Routledge is an imprint of the Taylor & Francis Group, an informa business
First issued in paperback 2013
© 1951 Hans Schaer, Translated by R. F. C. Hull

The publishers have made every effort to contact authors/copyright holders
of the works reprinted in the *International Library of Psychology*.
This has not been possible in every case, however, and we would
welcome correspondence from those individuals/companies
we have been unable to trace.

These reprints are taken from original copies of each book. In many cases
the condition of these originals is not perfect. The publisher has gone to
great lengths to ensure the quality of these reprints, but wishes to point
out that certain characteristics of the original copies will, of necessity, be
apparent in reprints thereof.

British Library Cataloguing in Publication Data
A CIP catalogue record for this book
is available from the British Library

Relgion and the Cure of Souls in Jung's Psychology
ISBN 13: 978-0-415-20946-5 (hbk)
ISBN 13: 978-0-415-86878-5 (pbk)
Analytical Psychology: 12 Volumes
ISBN 13: 978-0-415-21124-6
The International Library of Psychology: 204 Volumes
ISBN 13: 978-0-415-19132-6

CONTENTS

LIST OF ABBREVIATIONS
USED IN FOOTNOTES

PT — Psychologische Typen (*Psychological Types*)

PR — Psychologie und Religion (*Psychology and Religion*)

WSL — Wandlungen und Symbole der Libido (*Psychology of the Unconscious*)

BZIU — Die Beziehungen zwischen dem Ich und dem Unbewussten (*Two Essays on Analytical Psychology*)

SPG — Seelenprobleme der Gegenwart (partly reproduced in *Contributions to Analytical Psychology* and *Modern Man in Search of a Soul*)

WS — Wirklichkeit der Seele (partly in *Modern Man in Search of a Soul*)

UES — Über die Energetik der Seele (*On Psychical Energy*, in *Contributions to Analytical Psychology*)

EJ — Eranos-Jahrbuch (mostly untranslated, but *EJ 1934* in *The Integration of the Personality*; *EJ 1935* and *1936*, enlarged edition, in the forthcoming *Psychology and Alchemy*)

TRANSLATOR'S NOTE

Readers familiar with German will probably be aware that a standing problem in the translation of psychological literature is the word "Seele". The word is used in a very wide sense in German, and does not appear to carry with it the nimbus of exclusively religious, metaphysical, or even transcendental implications which attach to the word "soul" in modern English usage. I do not know why this non-psychological overtone should exist in English, for "soul" is as native to us as "Seele" is to the German language; indeed they derive from the same Saxon root. Nevertheless the overtone is so marked that, in order to avoid it, English psychologists tend more and more to speak of the "psyche" and of "psychic" phenomena or processes, just as until recently the spoke of the "mind" and still speak of "mental" diseases. Although the word "psyche" is gradually establishing itself in German, it has not yet succeeded in ousting "Seele" from its position as the subject of psychological investigation, an ironic fatality which seems likely to overtake the "soul" in English-speaking countries.

In Jungian psychology, a conceptual and empirical distinction is made between "Seele" and "Psyche". "Seele" is defined as the "internal personality", "the way in which one behaves in regard to his internal psychic (psychische) processes; it is the inner attitude, the character that one displays towards the unconscious". "Psyche", on the other hand, is "the totality

I

of all psychic processes, conscious as well as unconscious" (Psychological Types, Definitions). *A further distinction is made between the "objective psyche" (the unconscious) and the "subjective psyche" (ego-consciousness).*

From this it is clear that whereas the term "psyche" would be legitimate in any context—since a given psychological fact, state or process must be either conscious or unconscious—"soul" denotes more a function of relationship, and is the "link" between the conscious personality and the unconscious. As such a link, it is technically known as the "anima" ("animus" in women). The broad distinction between soul and psyche is not at all easy to adhere to in practice, and the extended use of "Seele" in Jung's own writings shows both the force of linguistic habit and the impossibility of applying the above definitions consistently.

The author of the present book writes not primarily as a psychologist but as a theologian. His use of the word "Seele" far exceeds that of "Psyche", but to translate it mainly by the latter term, as is now customary in psychological literature, might perhaps impart too strong a psychological colouring to his thought. For a Christian theologian the "soul" is surely rather more of a personal and moral entity than it can be for the psychologist, who sees it constantly dissolving back into the collective psyche from which it arose, like a wave of the sea. At the same time this dissolution has its counterpart in the "transcendental" aspect of the soul; for in mystical experience the soul is held to dissolve in God. In a theological context these personal, moral, and yet transcendental aspects seemed in place, and the word "soul" has therefore been used except where the author himself has "Psyche".

It may be of interest to note that, even for the Greeks,

2

"psyche" had the same double signification. Etymologically, it is cognate with ψῠχω, to breathe, blow, freshen, and with ψῠχόω, to animate. Like the Latin anima *and the Sanskrit* atman,[1] *it is thought that psyche originally meant "breath", and as such denoted the universal animating principle of which each "embodied" —we could hardly say "individual" —soul partakes and into which it returns. Psyche had therefore a personal and an impersonal aspect in Greek thought, just as the* atman *had in Hindu philosophy. Concurrently with this concept of the "breath-soul", psyche was also conceived as the "ghost-soul", the "double" which is seen in a man's shadow or in his image in water, and which parts company with him at his death, to dwell independently somewhere among the shades, whence it may reappear to the living as a ghost or in their dreams. Psyche in this sense corresponds to the Indian "purusha". The notion of an "individualized" soul mysteriously inhabiting a man's body, immortal and yet somehow compounded of his essential qualities, is, in the West, a relatively late product of philosophical speculation and was developed largely under Christian influence. The precise constitution of the soul is still a subject of theological controversy.*

[1]*It is a remarkable fact that the term "self" should reappear in Jungian psychology, where it serves as a symbol for wholeness, for the synthesis of the conscious and unconscious elements in the personality, which is achieved through the process of individuation. The "self" is both this individuating process and the goal towards which the individuant is developing; it may thus fittingly be called an "entelechy", i.e., that which bears its goal within itself. The discovery of the "self" would therefore seem to be a direct continuation of the ancient quest for the entity of that same name in Indian philosophy: the* atman, *no longer conceived on the primitive level as "breath", but spiritualized into the Absolute Subject. Immersing himself by contemplation in this One Reality, the contemplative "knows himself", and recognizes that he and this "self" are one and the same, besides which there is no other. The empirical relations between the psychological "self" and the various aspects of the psyche have, I think, yet to be clarified.*

The ancient idea of that torrent of universal life which the early Greek thinkers called "psyche" cannot be better formulated than in the words of Heraclitus: "Though you travel in every direction you will never find the bounds of the soul, so deep is the logos of it". This saying of the "dark philosopher", some may think, is not without application to the Jungian concept of the collective unconscious. It, too, is advanced as the ultimate ground of explanation for all empirically observable psychic processes; but, precisely because it is such a ground, it necessarily remains without explanation, and unfathomable.

A further word is necessary as regards footnotes. While the titles of Jung's works referred to in the text are in English, the references in the footnotes are to the German or Swiss editions. The reason for this procedure is that a new, revised, Collected Edition of Jung's works is to be published by Routledge & Kegan Paul in this country, and in America by the Bollingen Foundation, New York. The essays and lectures contained in certain of the existing English editions are to be regrouped according to subject-matter and published under different titles; and the major self-contained works will presumably have new page numbers. In the present volume, most of the quotations have been retranslated from the revised German editions. It has therefore been thought advisable to retain the German references so as to avoid confusion when the Collected Edition finally appears. A list of the abbreviations used is given on page vi, together with the corresponding English titles as available at present.

INTRODUCTION

IN A book by J. Gebser,[1] the statement is made that the psychology of C. G. Jung, regarded scientifically, is the nearest approach to religion. "The future will show," he says, "whether this psychological *re-connexion* (*religio*) can give rise to a spiritual one; whether the scientific course of subjective knowledge can lead without a break to the world of objective faith, which moulds the heart. In the fact—for this much can now be said for certain—that it is no longer exclusively 'psychology' in the scientific sense intended by Freud, but can already lay claim to the title of a teaching concerning the soul, lies the significance of Jung's 'complex psychology.' " Gebser, probably quite rightly, is chary of seeing in Jung's psychology a new religion, but for him Jung has introduced man's religious need into psychology. He has amplified Freud's idea of libido, which on the positive plane worked out as life-instinct and on the negative as death-instinct, and the amplification resulted in the recognition of a religious instinct. Thereby Jung's view of the soul became what Gebser calls the nearest approach to religion. Gebser makes this judgement in a book that offers a conspectus of the results of modern research in physics, biology, and psychology; and thus unwittingly he points to the conclusion, or at least tacitly implies, that through the mouth of Jung modern psychology begins to speak as the knower and

[1] *Abendländische Wandlung*, p. 175 (1942).

5

interpreter of religion. This is an eventful change, because so far theology has seemed to have the monopoly of all scientific interest in religion, concerning itself with it from the point of view of revelation. Psychology, however, makes the soul the direct object of investigation, and thus willy-nilly approximates to religion. Jung was not the first to recognize that the investigator of souls must perforce be an investigator of religion as well, but he was the first to take this fact into account with all its consequences. Gebser's interpretation of his work bears witness to this.

Theologians have not concerned themselves with Jung's conclusions to the extent that one would expect, things being what they are. There is no doubt that people in theological circles take the liveliest cognizance of Jung's publications. But one can hazard the statement that he is "relished with circumspection," indeed with all too great a caution. Theologians for the most part do not venture to follow out his thought in practice. They do not even undertake the experiment of utilizing his ideas as, at least, scientific hypotheses, to prove how they would serve when applied to theological problems. They are aware of Jung, are interested enough in his work, but there it stops, and the interest carries with it no obligations. Of course, many of Jung's thoughts on religion in general and on particular questions of religious life today are not undisputed and still need checking; but on the other hand, it is well-nigh grotesque that theologians should pretend that Jung's psychology simply does not exist or is in any case utterly unsuited to religious problems. These strictures apply not only to Catholic theology but more especially to Protestant. Jung himself says that his writings were at one time thoroughly studied and worked over in Catholic circles, while as yet no Protestant theologian had taken the trouble even to look into his works.[2] This state of affairs seems to have remained radically unchanged up to the present. Jung, who in his own words counts himself a left-winger in the parliament of Protestantism, yet finds more understanding with Catholic than with Protestant theologians. The reasons underlying this fact cannot be explained here, but it must be stressed. At the same time, there is among Protestant theologians no absolute lack of interest in psychology. It is exiguous enough, but it exists. The really astonishing thing is that Protestant theologians follow Freud's principles rather than Jung's, though Freud certainly does not make it easy for anyone with religious interests to approach religion through psychology. Nevertheless, when Protestants do apply the principles of psychology to the cure of souls, they give preference to Freud, despite the fact that in theory he repudiates religion and seeks to overcome it, while Jung has become more and more engrossed in religion and its psychic problems.

Professor Adolf Keller is to my knowledge the first Protestant theologian who has attempted to give a thorough and comprehensive account of Jungian psychology with reference to religion and the cure of souls.[3] "Through Jung's spiritual works there runs a peculiar, closely knit religious dialectic," he writes, "an almost inaudible communing with the Unknown. Now we hear the 'Yes' more distinctly, now the 'No.' The problem of religion has gradually acquired a ubiquity in Jung's thought that has no need of words to make itself felt. Where there is soul there is also religion—not, however, in the sense of an accepted ecclesiastical form, but of a

[2] *Die Beziehungen der Psychotherapie zur Seelsorge*, p. 10.
[3] *Die kulturelle Bedeutung der komplexen Psychologie*, Berlin, 1935.

7

fate-like encounter with a stronger spiritual reality which compels examination. If religion as generally understood rests on one's capacity to let oneself be profoundly affected by powers that transcend consciousness, then the first and essential thing about it is this influence and not the intellectual formulation of such experiences; for the formulation is bound to be made *a posteriori* on a plane that is alien to them. The reality of these seizures is prior to the truth of their conscious formulation. Jung has once more made room for this reality in psychology."[4]

These words, written about ten years ago, put the right interpretation on Jung's work. On religion proper Jung has to all appearances produced only one small book, called *Psychology and Religion*, which occupies a modest place in Jung's writings as a whole. We must not, however, let ourselves be deceived by appearances, for actually everything Jung has published has to do with religion to a greater or less degree. This is as true of his early large volume, *Psychology of the Unconscious*, as of his last, to be published under the title of *Psychology and Alchemy*. All are mines of information as regards the psychology of religion. No matter where you open Jung's psychology, you will always find flashes of insight and ideas that touch on the religious side of things, be it religion as a whole, or individual features of religious life, or finally the aberrations and pathological symptoms of religion.

The theologian who gets absorbed in Jung will be astonished again and again at the formidable and comprehensive knowledge Jung possesses both of Christianity and of the religions outside it. In this respect his knowledge is unique. Very few theologians or laymen

[4] *Ibid.*, p. 271.

have so wide a knowledge of religious life in all its forms as Jung has. He never gives you the impression that his explanations are just the ingenious flukes of a writer who is interested in everything and therefore also in religion, but who uses interesting presentation as a substitute for depth of thought. Even those who cannot agree with all Jung's interpretations must needs acknowledge his right to treat of religion, since his knowledge in this field is fundamental.

Not that Jung has as it were discovered religion for psychology. Psychoanalysis has studied it very intensively indeed, and this is true not only of Freud himself but of his pupils and fellow workers. Many of their publications are on religious subjects, and in the journal *Imago* psychoanalysis has provided itself with an organ designed to make public numerous psychological studies ranging over all the fields of cultural life, particularly religion. Following the example of Freud, however, most psychoanalysts view religion with a jaundiced eye and are of the opinion that although religion may indisputably have had a certain significance in the spiritual evolution of mankind, it no longer bears any relation to man's present psychic state and had better be dropped overboard. In this respect Freud is a representative of the view that prevailed among scientists in the nineteenth century, more especially the champions of the physical sciences. From the physical sciences this view insinuated itself into medicine, and thence via psychiatry into psychology. As is well known, Freud made a thorough study of French psychiatry under Charcot in Paris and under Bernheim in Nancy. This psychiatry had extensive dealings with religion on the principle that every pathological phenomenon is the exaggeration of a normal, healthy function. Accordingly, it was argued, you have in pathology normal phenomena writ large. Thus the French psychiatrists studied the pathological forms of religion and drew their own conclusions as to the value and significance of religion in general, with the result that they were more and more driven to the view that religion is an aberration of man's psychic life or at least but a stage in his spiritual development to be surpassed with all possible speed. If you accept the axiom that everything pathological is an exaggeration of the normal and apply it to religion, it is obvious that a conclusion of this kind is inevitable.

This basic rejection of religion determined for a long time the attitude of any psychology born of psychiatry. Through Leuba it was assimilated into the American psychology of religion. William James did not exactly adopt this attitude, though his great work *Varieties of Religious Experience* is clearly influenced by it; and psychoanalysis of the classical type represented by Freud has not as yet discovered any other attitude to religion. The verdict of the French school of psychiatry seemed all too well founded. Freud and his pupils also took over the procedure of employing pathological material as a basis for the assessment of normal phenomena. In most psychoanalytic writings we find observations made by the psychotherapist on neurotic individuals side by side with religious material, Christian or otherwise. The parallels thus displayed have all the appearance of exact correspondence; and since neurosis is a state of psychic sickness that can be overcome, religion is judged in like manner. This procedure was, with few exceptions, practised without scruple by the advocates of psychoanalysis for a long time. They did so with all the greater conviction since they knew that they were conforming to the scientific tendencies of their age. The victorious march of science, particularly the physical sciences, allowed them to hope that all the great problems of the world would be solved in due course, and thus there seemed to be no longer any place for religion, which was regarded as a primitive attempt to explain things. Accordingly they looked forward to its conquest and elimination by the continued progress of science; and the Freudian school of psychology believed it could make a substantial contribution to that end. There is, however, one exception to the psychoanalytic rule in matters of religion, and that is Dr. O. Pfister, of Zürich. Dr. Pfister is at once Protestant theologian and practising pastor on the one hand, and on the other a psychoanalyst in the strictest Freudian sense. It says much for the inner integrity of this man that he is able to take up an exceptional position in both fields. As against a psychoanalysis inimical to religion he defends the rights and values of religion; and as against a Protestant theology largely antipathetic to psychology he sets up Freud's teachings and defends them as an instrument of religious research and an important auxiliary in the cure of souls. It is obvious, therefore, that he is doing valuable pioneer work which merits the greatest respect. He has also rendered fine service in his researches into the pathological phenomena of religious life and brought much important material to light. He gives a fundamental lead in determining which are the deviations in religion that occur through psychic disturbances.

But despite all one's appreciation of his merits, a certain lack of unity is to be detected in Pfister's use of psychology, which is also apparent in his last big book, *Das Christentum und die Angst* (Christianity and Anxiety). This lack of unity arises from two factors, which are really interdependent. Firstly, he sees in psychoanalysis above all a method, and a method of cure, which undoubtedly it can be, though it is not exclusively that; but he fails to see it as a new, scientific, and broadly human form of *questioning*. Secondly, he never makes quite clear the ultimate rationale of Freud's judgements on religion. He enlists the aid of psychology to interpret the pathological forms of religion which seem questionable to him as a theologian. He sees in psycho-analysis a means for brushing aside any psychic obstacles that may block the individual's approach to what, according to Pfister's theological principles, constitutes the right religious outlook. But at this point Pfister thinks he has exhausted the possibilities of psychology. He does not call on it to give a deeper interpretation of those religious phenomena which cannot, in view of the history of religion and the Church, simply be written off as pathological, strange as they may appear to a Protestant. Further, he never tackles the question whether the motive principle of all scientific psychology—the urge to deeper self-knowledge—may not itself have a religious significance. Had he tackled these two points he would have seen in psychology more than the mere psychoanalytical techniques of psychotherapy, and would undoubtedly have clarified his position as regards Freud. Sooner or later he would have hit upon the truth that the construction Freud puts on many religious phenomena is rooted in Freud's own philosophy and view of the soul; and this might have led him to a radical examination of Freud's teachings on the latter subject, which would have shown up their rationale and their limitations. But having omitted to do this, Pfister has always handicapped his work with fragments of Freudian philosophy, which is by and large unsuited to religious interpretation. It is likely, too, that Freud himself did not base his philosophy on a thorough-going investigation of the whole phenomenon of religion and its values. This procedure, however, forces Pfister to employ psychology in a dualistic manner where religion is concerned. At one moment he makes consistent and incisive use of psychoanalytic principles, but when the psychologist in him runs the risk of coming into conflict with his theological *alter ego* he takes psychoanalysis only as a method, not a complete system of knowledge with its own definite views of life and the world. Hence that disunity and duality in his work, which probably explains why Pfister has always remained an exception in the Freudian school as regards the positive value he attributes to religion. Freud, of course, stuck faithfully to his original rejection of religion, and the great majority of psychoanalysts followed him in this.

For fairness' sake it must be added that though such systems of psychology as were not born of psychiatry or psychoanalysis have accepted religion and defended it, the results in these cases have not been very convincing. Academic psychology went its traditional way obsessed with definitions, abstract formulations, and theories, and these led to contradictions and schisms that effectively screened man and the living soul from the purview of the psychologist. For all that, the experimental psychology stemming from modern science had the appearance of trying to correct this lack of human perspective. But as applied to religion, it failed to impart much prestige to psychology in this direction. When one reads the *chef d'œuvre* of experimental psychology, Karl Girgensohn's *Der seelische Aufbau des religiösen Erlebens* (The Psychic Structure of Religious Experience), one is far from having the impression that religion has been plumbed to the depths. Despite the great scope of the book, which says much for the industry of the author who put it together, the net result is small. One seems to have heard already what is said here of the psychic structure of religious experience. It has all been said before by every dogma, by all the better books of religious devotion; and it is difficult to rid oneself of the suspicion that the outcome of the many lengthy and wearisome experiments was in reality established from the very beginning. A psychology of this kind was powerless to invalidate the results and conclusions of psychoanalysis. For psychoanalysis could always lay claim to two important points: it derived its material from living people, and it acquired it by a method whose legitimacy rested on the fact that it was able to heal those suffering from ills of the soul. Thus there appeared to be something true about it, and it is hardly surprising if psychoanalysts were but little impressed by the objections of other branches of psychology in matters of religion. If their conclusions were to be questioned, the problem would have to be tackled at a deeper level.

One other fact must be laid to Freud's credit. If he asserted that religion was an illusion without a future and must be replaced by a knowledge that was true to reality, he had in fact found material that could rightly be interpreted only in this way. Even outside psychoanalytical circles there are many people today who are profoundly convinced of the fallibility and questionableness of existing religious forms. Freud himself, as a Jew, knew that the Jewry of his time was changing, and in addition his medical practice acquainted him with Viennese Catholicism, of which it can safely be said that it offered no very sympathetic or persuasive example either of Catholicism or, for that matter, of Christianity. There were all sorts of decadent features which might easily convince an unbiased observer that the days of such a religion—or, better, religiosity—were numbered. And his international clientele familiarized him with typical examples of the Victorian Age, both English and Continental—an age which in the sphere of religion and ethics was endeavouring to infuse new life into perished formulae. If Freud recognized the hollowness of this undertaking, that only speaks in his favour. All that has happened since then proves to the hilt how shallow the effect of these efforts has been: had the Victorian Age really reached its goal, we would have been spared two World Wars. So that the unprejudiced judge must admit that Freud found for his pronouncements on religion objective material that admits of no other interpretation, and that he has said absolutely the right thing about certain forms of religiosity. But this material is far from covering all the phenomena of religious life, either of today or of the past. Moreover, it is a dubious procedure to apply these discoveries, which were based on particular forms of religion, themselves conditioned by the times, to religion in general. Above all, neither Freud nor the psychoanalytic school in the narrow sense has ever asked whether it might not be true that the neurotic person practises the forms and customs of religion in a morbid way, while the forms and customs themselves have quite another meaning. In the delight of the discoveries which the psychoanalytic method opened out to him, the investigator overlooked this problem. He examined religion and the world of myths according to strictly Freudian principles and thought he possessed the key to truth.

Such was the situation in psychology with regard to the place and the interpretation of religion that Jung met at the very outset of his work as psychiatrist and psychotherapist. On the one hand, there was keen criticism of religion, in many cases amounting to outright rejection. The material brought forward in corroboration of this point of view was weighty enough, since it came from men living in our time. It was not the product of mere curiosity or of fundamentally questionable experimentation, but had been given direct to the physician by spiritually sick persons who were looking for a cure. That this material had been rightly interpreted seemed proved by the fact that the interpretation went hand in hand with a medical technique of healing, which seemed to be vindicated in practice by the curative results. On the other hand, religion was approved, but more on the ground of theoretical considerations and in conjunction with psychological methods whose practical reliability was extremely doubtful and which could never compete in importance with those of psychoanalysis.

At the beginning of his work Jung had associations with Freud and collaborated with him. But this collaboration extended only to psychotherapy in the narrower sense. Philosophically, and in regard to religious questions as well as to the basic problems of psychic reality, Jung has remained true to the direction his development originally took before he ever came into contact with Freud. At all events, his publications show that he is far more cautious than Freud in his pronouncements on religion, and has always been so. Though he is wholly unprejudiced he takes religion with the utmost seriousness as a phenomenon of man's psychic life, and finds himself unable to discredit it merely for the sake of certain philosophical premises. But he is also aware of the many questionable factors in the field of religion, and whoever reads Jung knows that by no means everything that purports to be the highest manifestation of the human spirit or direct revelation from God can really be accepted as such. In this Jung is clearly following the lead of William James, whose aim was to build up a psychology *and* a pathology of religious life. Religion may be of the greatest importance to mankind, but the strangest instincts and aspirations can still find room in it. That is why religious life is such a pregnant subject of research for Jung, and why he uses his whole scientific equipment to bring to light its significance for man's psychic life. At the same time he points out the diversity of aims and motives that may reveal themselves in religion.

Jung does not confine his observations to Christianity but has a positive attitude to all religions and tries to do justice to them.[5] For the investigator who really wants to serve science, that is the only possible attitude. Jung takes each religion for what it is and never attempts to set up an *a priori* criterion and assert the truth of one and the untruth of all the others. If a religion is the living experience of a people or community or even of a single individual, it has justified its existence, and one has to accept it as such and give it due honour. In this respect, Jung is refreshingly free from prejudice compared with many theological inquirers. One of the interesting consequences of this is that Jung has a much clearer idea than most other scientists of the relations between Christianity and the non-Christian religions. He can compare them impartially both as they are now and as they were in the past, and one has the impression that he wants to be, and to a large extent is, fair to both. A similar impartiality is to be found, perhaps, only in Albert Schweitzer. Be that as it may, Jung has assembled

[5] *SPG*, p. 80.

a formidable mass of material—for instance, in his *Psychology of the Unconscious*—pointing to affinities between early Christianity and the religions of the last days of antiquity. What he has there collected in the matter of parallels respecting symbols, rites, dogmas, and myths is, quite apart from the psychological insight displayed, extremely impressive; so that the reader is likely to find an unexpected key to many of the historical problems of Christianity.

To many readers of Jung's writings, particularly those with a theological education, it may seem strange at first that one can search Jung in vain for a definition of religion corresponding, perhaps, to Schleiermacher's famous formula about religion's being "the feeling of utter dependence." This seeming omission, however, is not without its good reasons; for it is impossible to reduce all the phenomena of religious life to a simple formula. Either the formula will be taken in a very wide sense, in which case it is nugatory, or it will be coined with respect to one particular religion, in which case all the others are excluded from the field of observation or are regarded at the outset as untrue or imperfect approximations to the true one, so that one has made it impossible for oneself to do them justice. In all psychological, and indeed historical, research into religion, it is only right not to fix on any one definition, which is bound to be somewhat prejudiced. What alone serves the purpose is a purely formal description of such factors as one wishes to include in the field of observation.

If one inquires of Jung what the factors are that he counts as belonging to religion, one will find the following formulations: religion is the careful and scrupulous observation of the numinous.[6] "I want to make clear,"

⁶ *PR*, p. 12; pp. 15 f.

he says, "that by the term 'religion' I do not mean a confession of faith. It is true to say that every creed was originally based in part on the experience of the numinous, and in part on *pistis:* that is to say, trust, loyalty to and faith in a certain experience of numinous agencies, and in the change of consciousness that ensues; the conversion of Paul is a striking example of this. We might say, then, that the term 'religion' means the special frame of a mind that has been changed by experience of the numinous. The various creeds are the codified and dogmatized forms of original religious experience." Jung sees the meaningful and comprehensive nature of these experiences as a further characteristic of religion. "When a problem is taken religiously, it means, psychologically speaking, that it is taken as something very significant, of particular value, as something that affects the whole of a man and therefore also the unconscious (the abode of the gods, the Beyond, etc.)." [7] Another characteristic of religion is absoluteness: "An absolute attitude is always a religious attitude, and at whatever point a man becomes absolute, there you will find his religion." [8] Because of this absoluteness it is impossible to discuss religious experience. Either one has had it, and then one understands what it is all about, or else one has never experienced anything of the kind, and then this field is inaccessible and all discussion futile. Jung says: "I must point out that it is not a question of faith at all but of experience. Religious experience is absolute, and cannot be disputed. One can only say that one has never had such an experience, whereupon one's opponent will reply, 'Sorry, but I have.' It makes no difference what the world thinks about religious experience; those who have had it possess a great store of

[7] *PT*, p. 274.   [8] *SPG*, p. 207.

something that can be a source of life, meaning, and beauty for them; something that sheds a new radiance on the world and all men. Such people have *pistis* and peace." [9] Hence Jung cites only the following as marks of religious experience: its kinship with experience of the numinous, its absoluteness, and its quality of wholeness, that is to say, its connection with a man's personality taken as a whole.

On account of this last characteristic, Jung does not recognize a religious function comprising only one part of the soul, but he regards this function as being connected with the entire field of the psychic, with man's whole personality. Consequently, it is impossible to find one's bearings with regard to religion in Jung's psychology without first coming to terms with the whole structure of psychic reality as it appears there. We shall therefore concern ourselves in our first chapter with his psychology in a broad sense before venturing on the special questions of our theme.

[9] *PR*, pp. 188 *et seq.*; cf. p. 91.

ELEMENTS OF JUNGIAN PSYCHOLOGY

JUNG's psychology does not say: man has a soul or psyche. It says rather: man, as a psycho-physical being, partakes of psychic reality, or even: he is a part of psychic reality.[1] The moment you start on Jung's psychology you have the feeling of entering into a spacious new world that contains wide tracts of unknown territory and many secrets, and that accordingly holds out all sorts of possibilities of discovery. This new world is the world of the soul or the psychic, these terms being understood in their broadest sense. Just as the physical world known to us in modern science—in physics and chemistry on the one hand and astronomy on the other—extends into the infinitely great and the infinitesimally small without our having been able as yet to reach the limits of physical reality, so Jung presents the world of the psychic as infinite in extension. He abandons the old view according to which man is provided with a monad-like soul, and posits a psychic reality that is immensely extended, a reality in which the individual participates but which goes far beyond his consciousness. And just as no sharp line can be drawn in modern physics between man and the surrounding world, because the border-line is fluid, so the human soul cannot, for Jung, be sharply marked off from psychic reality, since the border-line is equally indistinct. A sharp division is as impossible here as between

[1] Wilhelm-Jung: *The Secret of the Golden Flower*, p. 122.

the human body and the atmosphere that surrounds it.

This standpoint of Jung's is sure to be somewhat astonishing for many people, because the argument as to whether the soul exists at all is still going strong. We have long taken it for granted that man has a soul. But the materialism of the nineteenth century, which even now seems to many people a very simple and therefore conveniently handy philosophy, denied the existence of the soul outright. Though many of them regarded this as an extreme view which they could not accept, they still entertained the idea popular for hundreds and thousands of years that the soul is a monad, that is, a self-enclosed unit. Further, they equated soul with consciousness. The human soul appeared as a tiny point exposed to the infinity of the universe, and this universe seemed to contain nothing of soul apart from man on this planet of ours. If the incidence of physical matter in the universe was something of a rarity, the incidence of soul was rarer still; and therefore—such was the conclusion even of those who were enemies of materialism—soul was of very small importance. When they spoke of reality they meant palpable and demonstrable reality, hence physical reality. They might not go so far as to deny the soul all reality and actuality, but they conceived it to be entirely dependent on the physical, even though the question of the connection between the physical and the psychical could never be carried to a satisfactory conclusion. The soul was localized in the brain, and they tried to localize the psychic functions in the brain's anatomy, on the assumption that cerebral processes were the cause and substantial basis of the psychic. Psyche seemed a mere by-product of physical processes, and these latter alone were accorded the character of reality. In the resultant cleavage between physical and psychic phenomena reality was attributed only to *physis*, while psyche was rated as imagination and meaningless appearance. When it came to acknowledging the world of the mind and art and science, the foundation of all this was still physical reality. The idealists, who believed in a spiritual world apart from the physical one and attributed as much or more reality to it, were always suspected as dreamers and devotees of delusion.

This outlook, which one took as a matter of course and which seemed to require no proof for the simple reason that one had been brought up in it, was vehemently contested by Jung. With a revolutionary will of almost Copernican proportions he set about building the world on an entirely new basis. In his view the question of psycho-physical relationship is insoluble today,[2] but what he does maintain is that the psychic is reality, i.e. is real (actual) because it *acts*. The reality of it is no whit inferior to that of the physical in significance, intensity, and extent. Nor can it be thought of as a mere appendage of physical existence, but it is grounded and complete in itself. Just as physical reality has its laws, forces, causes, and goals of development, so the psychic has its own energy, its own course of life, its own causes and purposes.

Wirklichkeit der Seele (Reality of the Soul) is the title of one of Jung's books, and in this can be seen a dominant theme in all his researches and writings. He is never tired of stressing again and again that *when a thing is psychic, it is at the same time pre-eminently actual.* Suppose someone is intensely concerned about a dream he had the previous night, Jung warns against saying: the dream is merely psychic and therefore without significance. On the contrary, he would say: the dream

[2] *UES*, pp. 14 *et seq.*

23

as a psychic fact is in the highest degree actual and therefore real. For Jung adopts the view that we never experience physical reality immediately, but only psychic reality. What we learn of the surrounding world we experience through our own soul. We have no immediate knowledge of physical reality; all we have are replicas of it in the soul. We never see the *Ding an sich*, only the pictures evoked by it within.[3] Our sensations, perceptions, and experiences are psychic data released by physical reality; hence the latter is never an immediate datum for man. Every so-called physical experience is at once psychic experience. There can be psychic experience without any simultaneous physical process to release it; but there can never be experience of physical processes in which psychic ones are not also at work. Therefore the physical world is never immediately given, but only the soul; and the only thing that is immediately accessible to us is the imagery of the soul.[4]

Consequently for Jung it is erroneous to try to explain psychic facts in terms of the physical. Such explanations are beside the point, for the soul is a reality in itself, independent of the physical.[5] No more than we can derive the physical world from anything else can we derive the soul from anything else. Hence psychology, as science, must regard everything to do with the soul as psychic reality which can be interpreted only in its own terms and cannot be derived from anything extraneous. Nor has psychology to demonstrate what is the purpose of the soul, any more than any other science can do this in respect of its subject. Psychology is a science in its own right and is moulded by its subject, the soul in the widest sense of the word; hence it must employ the methods appropriate to its subject. It falls short of its

[3] *SPG*, p. 383. [4] *Ibid.*, p. 183. [5] *UES*, pp. 14 *et seq.*

24

goal if it seeks to reduce the soul to something else—instinctual drives, for instance.

Since soul is the only immediate datum of experience, psychology is in the last analysis a highly problematical science. All knowledge is full of problems, because we are always faced with the question: what *is* perception of the surrounding world and what part of my perceptions rests on the data of my soul? As we all know, modern science is keenly aware of this problem and is obsessed with epistemology. The same problem is particularly urgent for psychology because it is knowledge of the soul, and this knowledge can come only through the soul. In our experience of the psychic we experience primarily our own soul, even when we are concerned with psychic life outside ourselves. We import into the other person what we have in ourselves. This importing cannot be altogether unjustified if the structure of the other person corresponds to our own. But this is not established *a priori* and, as experience shows, is very often not the case. Most people are naïve enough to think that they can have their say in psychological matters, and yet their sort of psychology is simply the psychology of their own soul. But it is not only the layman who carries his own psychology over into the psychic life outside him: it also happens with scientifically minded psychologists. Thus Jung shows that Freud's psychology is conditioned by the psychological type that Freud was, Freud's attitude being obviously extraverted. Adler, on the other hand, whose psychology is so different from Freud's that many think they must choose either the one or the other and can never combine both, wrote the psychology of the introvert, because he probably belonged to this type. So it is not only the ordinary "student of human nature" who naïvely imposes his own brand of psychology on others; it is the scientists as well. Both are faced by the fact that experience of their own soul and of the psychic life extraneous to it comes to them in an almost indissoluble combination.

It is understandable, therefore, why psychology appeared so late and is thus a very young science. For it demands a certain degree of consciousness to recognize the reality of the soul. We live in and through the soul and are so wrapped up in it that we do not notice it at all. It is—in the Kantian sense—a phenomenon. To recognize the difference between the thing-in-itself and the thing-as-it-appears requires a degree of psychic consciousness and differentiation which mankind only reaches quite late and which is by no means given to all even today.

If, then, the reality and range of the soul are being discovered today, this discovery is connected with our spiritual life as a whole: the hour for such a knowledge has struck. The fact that the dark womb of the soul contains more than has been suspected up to the present is a realization that is slowly dawning on our spiritual horizon and that has been growing clearer ever since Kant, who had some inklings of it in his philosophy. The romantic and physician C. G. Carus also felt it, likewise Schopenhauer, J. J. Bachofen, and, more vividly, Nietzsche. Today our knowledge of the external world has reached a stage where inquiry turns inwards to the domain of the soul. The physicist's knowledge that, objectively speaking, there are no colours but only vibrations, and that colour-perception takes place only in the individual, is not without bearing, since it is patent that something interposes itself between individual and object, or that the individual perceives his surroundings only through a medium, which is the soul. Furthermore, this intensive preoccupation with the soul was stimulated by medical science. In the nineteenth century this was really concerned only with the human body, but the thorough knowledge of it that resulted from this one-sidedness turned the attention of medical men to the soul. They found the soul to be a cause of sickness, recognizing the psychic basis of mental diseases; and then the studies of French psychiatrists on such subjects as hysteria, hypnosis, and suggestion first pointed the way to possible cures through psychic means. Freud and Breuer built these beginnings up into a new branch of medical science, thanks to their painstaking investigations, which afforded psychology the practical and theoretical prerequisites for intensive work. So that empirical knowledge and the need to heal the sick both point to the soul as something actual and alive. The soul is *the* problem of modern man; and Jung's aim is to make a psychological synthesis of all the knowledge we have so far acquired in the various fields by various methods of research. He is perhaps the first to set out to build a theory of the soul that takes account not only of "professional psychology" but also of religion, mythology, alchemy, art, and literature.

If the soul is real, if, that is to say, it *works,* then it must be life, a living process, a living event. In Jungian psychology we can never see the soul as something finished and rounded, or a psychic fact as something constant and static: soul is always alive and happening. Just as modern science resolves all physical data, matter included, into motion and events, so Jung does with the soul. The process had already started with Freud when he associated the soul very closely with instinctual life, hence with something dynamic. Jung loosens this tie with the instinctual drives to a large extent, but stresses all the more the livingness of the soul, pointing

27

out again and again that it is in process, movement, development, always happening, never stiff and dead. From this he has taken the inferential step of establishing the idea of psychic energy—libido. Just as there is energy in physics, so there is energy in psychology. Freud likewise used the idea of libido, but he meant sexual drives. Jung extends it to psychic energy. "By libido I understand psychic energy," he says. "Psychic energy is the *intensity* of the psychic process, its psychological value. By this I do not mean to imply any imparted value, whether moral, aesthetic, or intellectual; the psychological value is simply conditioned by its *determining* power, which expresses itself in definite psychic operations ('effects'). Neither do I understand libido as a psychic *force*, a misunderstanding that has led many critics astray. I do not hypostasize the concept of energy, I only employ it as a term for intensity or value. The question as to whether or not a specific psychic energy exists has nothing to do with the concept of libido. Often I use the terms 'energy' and 'libido' quite promiscuously." [6] Psychic energy can, for example, work out mainly as sexual instinct—when it is strongly sexualized. It can be turned primarily to the external world, thus giving rise to the extraverted attitude; or it can turn more inwards as in introversion. It can drive an individual forward to the realization of new tasks, plans, objectives—progression; or, if the individual shrinks from tackling problems that he feels are beyond him, it can recede to such an extent that he gets stuck at a point in his development which he should have overcome—regression. In the last resort regression means trying to conquer a new situation by recapitulating an old one to which one feels equal. But it can also consist in reducing the scope of one's

[6] *PT*, p. 645.

life and confining the libido to just a few objects, because one failed when one spread one's interests and one now lacks self-confidence. In normal circumstances libido is bound up with our interests and attention, hence with the sphere of consciousness. It can, however, fall into the unconscious and so energize the unconscious functions that little of it is left over for consciousness. In this state consciousness is paralyzed, while the unconscious is full of tensions which may seek easement in wholly unexpected ways, in real explosions.

Jung uses the idea of libido instead of that of will. We shall see in due course that the will does not appear among the four basic functions that Jung enumerates. Will is *purposive libido;* and he chooses the term "libido" because in cases of paralysis of will psychic energy is still present and may powerfully engage the individual's attention. Since libido is the more comprehensive idea and can thus cover unconscious phenomena as well, whereas will is always bound up with consciousness, Jung prefers "libido" to "will." Whatever is infused with libido is psychically active and makes itself felt, either creatively or, in the case of psychic disturbances and illnesses, obstructively and inhibitingly. We must realize, however, that the individual cannot control his libido at will; on the contrary, it can withdraw from consciousness and then prove stronger than all our reasons. Nor can it, as energy, be switched on and off; rather, it must be likened to a river which can, within limits, be controlled and led in a certain direction but which will always display an inner law of its own that has to be reckoned with. Libido is always at one remove from the conscious mind and its influence; and sometimes it does the very thing one does not want and does not expect. In this respect the soul shows itself to be irrational, greater than consciousness, greater than life as ordinarily understood.

This can be seen more clearly when we come to the question of the *extent* of the psychic sphere. Jung, true to his view that soul is not made up of monads but is a reality in its own right, gives it unlimited extension. Man has a wide experience of psychic data; he has thoughts and ideas, dreams and fantasies, and the whole world of art, mythology, religion, even of politics and economics, belongs to the soul. In all these phenomena of human life the soul plays an active part and has its being in them. But it also has its being in such tremendous catastrophes as the two World Wars, where stirrings and impulses awaken in man that fill him with horror. The soul has a life that wrings our highest admiration from us; it has another life that sheds night and abysmal darkness around it and sends a chill down our spines. In all human relationships the soul lives and vibrates too, but soul is far from being something harmless and simple. What a man knows of revelation he knows through his soul, and through his soul too he knows the powers that destroy and annihilate.

So as to leave no room for misunderstanding it must be emphasized at once that Jung never equates soul with the ego and consciousness. Soul goes beyond the sphere of personality in the sense that by no means all the impulses a man feels within him can be ascribed to his ego. As St. Augustine has already said, a man cannot be held responsible for his dreams; similarly, there are other psychic contents which, though inwardly experienced, lie beyond the range of our personality. That is why personality has a range for Jung that was unknown in the earlier psychologies. Man has a consciousness which builds itself up round the ego-function. The ego is the centre of consciousness. A part of the personality, however, is not co-ordinated with this ego and not conscious; hence the soul extends into the unconscious. Consciousness is, figuratively speaking, only the tip of a cone whose base goes deep down into the unconscious realm; and this *personal unconscious* which lies comparatively close to the ego passes over into psychic territory that is no longer accessible to the individual. The unconscious is not a self-contained magnitude. If one may make use of an image, the individual personality is like an island rising out of the sea. Everything above water is bathed in the light of consciousness. But the whole rests on the sub-aqueous base of the island, on the unconscious; and this imperceptibly loses itself in the unfathomable depths of the ocean. Jung gives no definition of the unconscious except that it is an attribute of psychic processes which cannot be understood,[7] or the "Absolutely Other" of consciousness.[8] Jung has devoted the greater part of his research work to unconscious psychic functions and processes; his primary interest is with the unconscious, and, in contrast to the earlier psychologists, he only pursues the psychology of consciousness in conjunction with that of the unconscious.

The idea of the unconscious first appears in Carus's work, although professional psychology failed to take it up. Then Eduard von Hartmann worked with it in philosophy, and Freud assimilated it into his psychology. Jung has always disputed the Freudian idea of the unconscious very strongly. For Freud the unconscious is the place where a man deposits all the psychic contents that, for one reason or another, he is unable to understand, either because he lacks the time and strength, or

[7] *Analytische Psychologie und Erziehung*, p. 61.
[8] *SPG*, p. 366 n.

31

because the contents are somehow unpleasant and painful for him. According to Freud, it is the latter that make up the bulk of such unconscious contents, and they refer mostly to love-life in the widest sense of the word. Experiences of this kind are, as Freud says, "repressed." In the case of young people it is a matter of instinctual impulses that they do not know what to do with, or of shocks, or of stirrings in their own psyches which do not conform to the accepted moral standards and rules of life. In time they form a deposit of disagreeable memories and impulses which the person in question refuses to acknowledge but which he cannot forget despite all his efforts. Because he does not allow them to emerge into consciousness they make themselves felt in dreams, fantasies, everyday errors, symptoms, and complexes of all kinds that may lead to neurosis. The neurosis can be cured only if the repressed contents are made conscious.

Jung accepts this theory of Freud's for certain cases, though he does not stop there. In his view Freud's theory is valid primarily for neurotics in the early stages of life, who can in fact often be cured by having their repressions made conscious. But under the stress of his psychotherapeutic practice Jung saw himself compelled to give up the equation: unconscious equals repressed material. All repressed material is unconscious, but there are many other psychic contents and functions that are equally unconscious. Much of it never reaches the threshold of consciousness, for instance subliminal perceptions and memories of all kinds, particularly those of early childhood; latently developing changes of personality such as manifest themselves in religious conversions; and other factors which are played out in the unconscious. Therefore Jung thinks that the unconscious can never be exhausted by the conscious-making processes of analytical therapy, which would have to be assumed according to Freud's view.[9] Thus the unconscious has a greater range for Jung than for Freud.

Comparing Freud's, Jung's, and Carus's teachings concerning the unconscious, one soon remarks that Jung is nearer to Carus than is Freud. Carus begins his well-known work, *Psyche*, with the words: "The key to the knowledge of the nature of conscious psychic life lies in the region of unconsciousness." In sum, Carus says something like this: only that part of the soul is conscious which is connected with the ego. But this is only a small part of our human life. Carus denies the widespread idea that the essential thing in man is his spiritual personality and that the body is a negligible factor. For him life is a psychophysical unit. What we experience on the surface as body-world we experience underneath as psychic reality. Since there are many living processes in the body of which we are not conscious, consciousness is but a small part of psychic processes in general. The conscious mind therefore is only a small part of psychic reality; the rest is unconscious. But the unconscious is the vehicle, the basis of conscious psychic life, and for Carus consciousness is never explicable through itself but only through the unconscious. We can have unconscious life without consciousness, but never *vice versa*. He sees the unconscious as coinciding with that element in life which creates unconsciously; hence for him man, through the psychically unconscious, is rooted immediately in life. The life of the soul is to be compared to the ceaseless flow of a river which is lit up only in parts by the light of the sun, i.e. consciousness. "Long before we ever became conscious of the majority of our ideas

[9] *BZIU*, p. 11.

and feelings, the soul was living an unconscious life of great complexity." Carus knew that individual existence is not only nourished but also harassed by the dark instinctive forces of elemental life. The unconscious is not a low and unimportant stage in the development of ideas and knowledge, but the matrix of all our driving-forces, feelings, thoughts, actions.

Carus builds these ideas up into a metaphysical view of man. Man is the living and incarnate idea that rises from the ocean of unconscious life and realizes itself in it, achieves mind and wins to freedom from instinct but is always rooted in the unconscious. Jung does not go so far into metaphysics. He only wants to concern himself with psychology. Still, something of Carus's view of the unconscious is to be found in Jung. In his essay "Seele und Erde" [10] he tells us on the basis of his experience with American patients how these, being of European descent, ought, when they reproduce myth-material in their dreams, to draw on European mythology. But that is not the case. On the contrary, they employ themes from the myths of the Redskins and other native races. Therefore, Jung argues, the soul's unconscious functions are affected by the soil man lives on. He does not draw any further conclusions, but we are not very far from Carus's idea that through the unconscious we are linked to the life-process in all its forms.

Carus came to his ideas intuitively—Jung investigates the unconscious with all the scientific equipment of the modern physician. The things that Carus brought forward in baffling fragments only, Jung builds up into a new and wonderful world.

[10] "Mind and the Earth," in *Contributions to Analytical Psychology* (SPG).

To sketch Jung's view of the unconscious, one must begin with the thought that the unconscious has a meaning for real life that is at least equal to that of the conscious mind.[11] The conscious mind is never the soul itself, and the unconscious functions are as valuable as the conscious ones; they have a significance and sovereignty of their own. In what he does and leaves undone man is as much conditioned by them as by consciousness. Such statements may sound astonishing to the modern Western ear and seem like an absolutely new discovery. But the unconscious was always there, and if we did not know it, that was only because we could not know it or did not want to. We were not strong enough to come to terms consciously with the unconscious, were and still are afraid of it. And rightly—for the road to the unconscious is the road to darkness, to the unbounded, the nameless, where unknown experiences and terrors lurk. Also, it is a dangerous road for Western man, who has long concerned himself with consciousness only. Contact with the unconscious is an alarming procedure and not at all harmless, for it may well bring the danger of psychosis and insanity. Psychosis comes about through the flooding of consciousness with unconscious contents;[12] and by descending into the unconscious we draw these contents closer to consciousness. So that the European's dread of the unconscious is understandable enough, but on the other hand, it is beside the point to pretend that the unconscious simply is not there. In Jung's view it is an ineluctable necessity for Western man to acquaint himself with the unconscious today.[13]

A primary manifestation of the unconscious is fantasy-thinking such as is found among children and primitives.

[11] UES, p. 144.   [12] EJ 1935, p. 23.   [13] WS, pp. 88 et seq.

Directed thinking tries by experiment or mathematical calculation to establish the connexion between cause and effect. Primitive thinking, as in magic, starts with analogies and rests on a psychic state that Lévy-Brühl called *participation mystique*. In this, an inner connexion is assumed to exist in all things, and thus it should be possible to bring about physical changes by magic words. This feeling that all is one is based on a high degree of unconsciousness; hence the fantasy-thinking of primitives is the thinking of the unconscious.[14] We could call fantasy-thinking instinctive in so far as instincts give rise to typical forms of action which repeat themselves systematically.[15] We meet with such thinking among adult Europeans in certain circumstances, above all in dreams.

For Jung, dream and fantasy are the royal road to the unconscious, since they reflect unconscious processes. We do not actually perceive these processes in dreams—for in themselves they are inaccessible to us—but we perceive their reflexions. Through them we can see something happening in the unconscious, and by interpreting dreams and fantasies we come to know the inner workings of these processes. Thus we can get to know of the individual's changes of attitude. Consequently, Jung goes further than Freud in his interpretation of dreams. For Freud, dreams contain indications of repressed material and wish-fulfilments which are denied in real life. According to this, dreams would be expressions of the life-will whose unfolding is limited by life's needs.[16] Jung accepts this theory of Freud's for certain dreams, but is of the opinion that it is not valid for all. Dreams, he thinks, are expressions of a psychic activity which is spontaneous and beyond the reach of conscious voli-

[14] *WSL*, I, p. 144.   [15] *UES*, p. 195.   [16] *Ibid.*, p. 126.

tion.[17] In the dream the actual state of the unconscious expresses itself in symbolical form.[18] Dreams and visions arise through autonomous complexes: formations of psychic content dissociated from the ego and leading an independent life of their own.[19] Dreams give us pictures which are symbolical and thus not immediately accessible to our intellectual understanding, but must first be interpreted. The interpretation makes their content conscious. But uninterpreted dreams work just as much on the psyche as a whole even when they are not understood. The unconscious processes underlying the dream will accomplish themselves in any case; only, in the uninterpreted dream the effect of the deep-seated psychic event remains for the time being unconscious. [20] That certain important portions of the soul should remain unconscious is not, however, always compatible with psychic health, and then the dream must be interpreted, i.e., the meaning of the dream, which is of a phylogenetically older order, must be translated into our normal forms of thinking.[21]

There can be no lexicon of dream interpretation which would lay down a meaning for every conceivable kind of content. Fixed symbols exist, at most, only in the case of repressed material, as Freud shows them in his system of interpretation. But when the analysis has raised the repressed material to consciousness and the same dream-images still continue to appear, there must be something else at the back of it. In interpreting dreams one must always bear in mind the fact that the unconscious can express anything with anything.[22] Thus the sexual symbolism postulated by Freud may in fact refer to sexual impulses, but in many cases it expresses something quite

[17] *BZIU*, p. 18. [19] *Ibid.*, p. 207. [21] *Ibid.*, p. 129.
[18] *UES*, p. 157. [20] *Ibid.*, p. 124. [22] *SPG*, p. 312.

different. Jung holds that the dream must have a sensible and meaningful value for the dreamer if it has been interpreted rightly. If, however, the interpretation is not accepted by the dreamer, then either there is no confidence as between dreamer and analyst or the interpretation given is wrong. Only the concrete situation can show which is which.

Jung discovered in his psychotherapeutic practice that dream interpretation becomes more difficult if the analysis is protracted. Thus, in a case reported by him,[23] he observed that dream-contents which had already been interpreted obstinately persisted. If something apparently known for a long time keeps on being reproduced in the dreams, this indicates a stoppage of psychic development. There was the further difficulty that contents appeared for which no associations could be found in the life and experience of the dreamer. This situation was in the highest degree disconcerting for both dreamer and psychotherapist. The person being analysed was disquieted by the unintelligible dreams, for when dreams go on producing incomprehensible and obviously peculiar contents it is only understandable that he should take fright at the unknown drama being played out in his soul. Jung for his part was also helpless in such a situation and, after much misgiving, decided on a course that was as bold as it appeared simple—to continue the analysis. The result proved him right in this intuitive decision, for it disclosed a new point of view. He found out that these dreams, so baffling at first, contained analogies with mythological images and processes and that such material gave hints of a possible interpretation. So he began on a new interpretative method, namely the examination of whole series of dreams, amounting some-

23 *BZIU*.

times to several hundreds. If a dream fails to afford the dreamer any meaningful and satisfying interpretation of its own accord, then Jung tries to establish its context; that is, he urges the dreamer to give out all the ideas he may have regarding the dream as a whole and the individual elements of it ("amplification"). After that he tries interpreting the whole series and the single dreams reciprocally. In the *Eranos-Jahrbuch 1935* he presents fragments from such a series and their interpretation; he uses the same series in *Psychology and Religion*, and further excerpts appear in *Psychology and Alchemy*.

Jung distinguishes dream interpretation on the objective level and on the subjective level. Interpretation on the objective level assumes that the dream-figures refer to the dreamer's relationships with his surroundings. For instance, all the persons figuring in a dream so interpreted are taken as real people, not symbols. If they are not recognizable at first, the interpretation tries to bring out exactly who is meant by the dream. Interpretation on the subjective level takes the dream as the reflexion of psychic processes relating to the dreamer's inner world and not his surroundings. Thus, the figure of a woman is regarded not as representing a real person from the circle of the dreamer's acquaintance, but as the *anima* or soul-image (see below). In many dreams the practised psychologist can tell at once whether they must be interpreted on the objective or the subjective level. Other dreams, because of the ambiguity of the psychic event in question, appear meaningful to the dreamer only when interpreted in both ways. Interpretation on the subjective level is indicated in the second half of life.

Continued investigation of the unconscious obliged Jung to distinguish between the personal unconscious and the supra-personal or collective unconscious.[24] The personal unconscious is made up of the individual's memories and experiences and also of his repressions. It is the precipitate of a man's experience of life. Here, for instance, arises the feeling of inferiority, which indicates that an unconscious portion of the soul should be made conscious and assimilated. Analysis of the personal unconscious leads to deepened self-knowledge.[25] But in connexion with his work on dream-analysis Jung discovered that the digesting of personal memories and repressed material hardly exhausts the unconscious. The analysis can be stopped at that point, but with many patients Jung found it necessary to continue the analysis because, although the past had been clarified with the raising to consciousness of personal memories, there was a complete lack of orientation as regards the future. Jung tells in an almost amusing manner how he was forced to realize in the case of a woman patient that a Freudian analysis, which only brings out the contents of the personal unconscious, leaves the analysed person as it were in mid air at the critical juncture, because he sees no road into the future. That is why so many analyses come to grief: assimilation of the past fails to evoke a new orientation, and that alone constitutes healing. At first Jung had no idea what to say, for he was unwilling to afford the patient an answer to the most personal of human questions—the meaning of his or her own life.

In this case, either the patient would not have accepted the doctor's advice or, had she done so, would have become hopelessly dependent on him. Both results would have invalidated the treatment. The patient had to find out for herself the answer to her question about the meaning of her life. Since consciousness did not

[24] *Ibid.*, p. 26.   [25] *Ibid.*, p. 27.

yield it, Jung resolved on a further advance into the unconscious, which led to a fragment of psychic life emerging that could not be explained in terms of personal memory and clearly bore an archaic and mythical stamp. Jung interpreted it as the precipitate of the experience of all mankind, not only of the single individual. This he called the collective unconscious. Just as in the body-structure there are certain correspondences among men of all races and all ages, and just as the body contains vestiges of earlier stages of development, so there are certain correspondences in the soul between all men, including a precipitate of bygone evolutionary stages.[26] In the collective unconscious, therefore, we encounter the primordial images or *archetypes*.

Jung thus characterizes certain functional potentialities of the collective unconscious. The archetypes or primordial images cannot be logically understood; they are dominants of the collective unconscious, "patterns of behaviour"[27]—functional engrams in which the age-old experience of mankind is crystallized and which lead people into typical patterns of behaviour. "They do not consist of inherited ideas but of inherited predispositions to reaction."[28] For all practical purposes the archetypes might be called "self-portraits of the instincts." They are to be found in all religions, in all esoteric doctrines, mythologies, legends, fables, sagas;[29] but they can also occur even when their mythological character is not recognized.[30] It is always a question of psychic data and not of mere representations of external reality. Astrology, too, uses the archetypes, but projects them into the constellations of heaven.[31] Jung also calls

---

[26] *Ibid.*, p. 45.
[27] *Geleitwort und psychologischer Kommentar zum Bardo Thödol*, p. 27.
[28] *BZIU*, p. 139.

[29] *EJ*, 1934, p. 182.
[30] *UES*, p. 198.
[31] *EJ*, 1934, p. 182.

the archetypes the psychic aspect of the brain-structure; as such they are forms of adaptation and represent the chthonic portion of the soul.[32] They have a rather dubious and ambiguous character, in the same way that the world must always remain an enigma to man. There can be no final interpretation of the meaning of the world, and in their effects on us the archetypes are just as baffling and unpredictable. On their emergence into consciousness they may lead us to a higher existence, but they can also threaten us with schizophrenia.[33] The archetypes are always present in any reactions that exceed the normal.[34] At the same time they are a powerful agent in the evolution of mankind, for they compel man to act against nature, with the result that he does not forfeit his soul to her. They extricate him from the bonds of the natural process and constrain him to adapt himself to the psychic world.[35] In every compelling ideal the archetypes are at work, and the man who understands how to speak in archetypes can rouse the unconscious—and this is often more valuable than a purely intellectual attitude.[36] Poets speak powerfully in archetypes, and a good part of the effect of a work of art lies in this. The figure of Faust is a typical "primordial image."

In one of his latest publications [37] Jung has added a new element to the archetype: the "karma-factor." The Indian term *karma* refers to a certain aspect of the doctrine of metempsychosis, namely the influence exerted on a subsequent existence by what has happened in the previous existence. Popularly it is interpreted as the reward and punishment, in the next life, of actions performed in this life. Jung does not take over the doctrine of

[32] *SPG*, p. 179.
[33] *Bardo Thödol*, pp. 28 et seq.
[34] *SPG*, p. 179.
[35] *Ibid.*, p. 324.
[36] *Ibid.*, p. 70.
[37] *Über die Psychologie des Unbewussten.*

metempsychosis, but he sees the collective unconscious as containing remnants of ancestral life.[38] "Whereas the memory-images of the personal unconscious are, as it were, filled out, because personally experienced by the individual, the archetypes of the collective unconscious are not filled out because not personally experienced. On the other hand, when psychic energy regresses, going even beyond the period of early infancy, and breaks into the legacy of ancestral life, then mythological images are awakened: these are archetypes." Jung regards this aspect of *karma* as indispensable for a deeper understanding of the archetype.

Owing to their archaic character, the archetypes are drawn from the simplest human conditions. Thus there is the archetype of the mother, the father, meaning (personified as a magician), the divine maid, the divine child, etc. Being unconscious, they are, like all the other contents of the unconscious, projected, i.e. *read into*, the external world. Thus, when observing a certain object, we do not see it as it is in itself, but we see it together with what we read into-it. In this way our relations with our surroundings are modified. When, for instance, we read the mother-archetype into our real mother, our relationship is conditioned not only by her but also by the archetype, and is complicated. This may result in a mother-complex. The characteristics we then read into the real mother are not present in her at all; all that is needed is the bare possibility of projecting them into her. Every powerful human bond rests on the projection of an archetype, and the bond can be loosed only with the lifting of the projection. Either we transfer the libido attaching to this archetype on to another one, or we make the function of the archetype conscious. The

[38] *Ibid.*, p. 140.

43

transference of libido on to another archetype is the sole purpose of many primitive religious rites—e.g. that of initiation.

Neither archetypes nor the collective unconscious can, it must be stressed again, be understood in the concrete sense. They are functions of which we are not conscious, containing potentialities of certain definite reactions. Many people never get to know anything of these functional possibilities latent in themselves; others have to make them active in certain circumstances.[39] What happens in individual cases will depend on the psychic situation. The widespread penchant for anthroposophy, theosophy, and similar religious cults indicates in Jung's view that many people have a wish to experience these functions in one form or another.

In the dim bygone of human history all men lived in the collective unconscious. They lived in a state of common unconsciousness, the so-called *participation mystique*. Later man rose to greater consciousness and freed himself more and more from the darkness. Today it is operative only in dreams, fantasies, visions of typically archaic character which remind us of the various mythologies. Primitives, however, still have a distinct feeling that this collective unconscious exists, for they distinguish between "little" and "big" dreams.[40] They take all dreams seriously. But ordinary dreams concern only the individual, and these are the dreams of the personal unconscious. Big dreams are dreamt by none save the chief, the medicine-man, or the priest, and they are made known to everybody since they are of general significance. They are regarded as revelations, and their character shows that they come from the collective unconscious. The civilized man of today is helpless in the

[39] *BZIU*, p. 68.   [40] *Ibid.*, p. 100.

face of "big" dreams: he may have dreams that engage his attention, but even here he has no idea what to do about them.

We have already said that Jung grants the unconscious as great and significant a part in the life of the individual as his conscious mind. He does this because the unconscious is *compensatory* to consciousness. The two are related and mutually dependent; the function of the unconscious is compensation, not contrariety or contradiction.[41] The unconscious has the power of intervening and striking a balance when the attitudes adopted by consciousness are too extreme. For instance, if a man puts an unwarrantably high value on himself or others, the compensation may occur through dreams; or when consciousness lets any function drop, that function falls into the unconscious and makes itself felt from there—as conscience, perhaps.[42] Many who, as far as their consciousness goes, have effected a complete break with religion, have dreams with an obviously religious content. Thus, the unconscious activates those functions and attitudes which consciousness either allows to lapse or simply ignores. Thus one can never say in advance exactly what the unconscious is going to set functioning, though whatever it does set functioning will always have a meaning, and will tend to protect the individual from extremes or one-sidedness. In other words, the unconscious functions in such a manner as to establish the individual's wholeness. It thus makes an important contribution to personality.

Jung has investigated the significant nature of the unconscious still more closely and finds that it can think teleologically,[48] a fact of the greatest importance for

[41] *Ibid.*, p. 98.   [48] *PR*, p. 71.
[42] *Analytische Psychologie und Erziehung*, p. 51.

45

religion. The unconscious can reveal thoughts that would not have emerged to consciousness at all and are therefore extremely weighty.[44] It has the power of regulating the soul;[45] indeed, a healing of the soul can often come from it.[46] In this connexion I would refer back to the patient who could find in her conscious mind no answer to the question about her life's meaning, but for whom this burning problem was ultimately solved by the workings of the unconscious. When the conscious mind has lost its bearings, the advance into the unconscious can often bring about a new and meaningful direction of personality. This explains the fact, observed by many psychotherapists, that the dreams which some patients have before the first session contain clear indications of the individual's problem and the possibilities of curing it. Such dreams often run directly counter to consciousness, and a good deal of the analyst's work consists in making them intelligible and acceptable to the dreamer. It is not for nothing that the East, far more experienced in its dealings with the soul than the West, opposes our activism and purposefulness and recommends simply letting psychic life take its course. For in many cases this uninfluenced and unobstructed activity of the soul leads to a more valuable understanding than our fanaticism of will and consciousness ever can. As an interesting example of the meaningful workings of the unconscious, Jung refers to the preparations the soul makes for dying. He has come across cases where death announced itself while yet there were no signs of life coming to an end. But it was clearly indicated that the soul was preparing itself for death. Evidently it is not a matter of indifference to the soul

[44] *Ibid.*, p. 71.
[45] *BZIU*, p. 79.
[46] *Die Beziehungen der Psychotherapie zur Seelsorge*, p. 27.

how a man dies.[47] The end is announced in images of a new life, of change, or something of that kind. Carus's premonition that the unconscious creates life finds confirmation in Jung's psychology.

Jung has also seen cases of a supra-personal plane forming itself in the unconscious, from which there arose a new experience and intuition of God. We shall come back to this later, but can lay it down now that the unconscious is the seat of original religious experience. Even when personality has collapsed, the unconscious can take over the lead. We see this, for instance, in religious conversions like that of the apostle Paul. Certainly it must never be overlooked that such transformations and enlargements of personality are not by any means easy and without danger. The approach to the unconscious exposes the ego to the danger of disintegration. That is why a man descends into the unconscious only at a time of crisis for his soul; the coming to grips with these psychic forces is a hard and serious business which demands the application of the whole man. Nothing is more dangerous and imprudent than to provoke them unnecessarily, for in the last analysis the ego is weaker than the unconscious when this shows its destructive face.

From the foregoing it will be clear how much significance Jung attaches to the unconscious. It is not the appendage or dumping-ground of the conscious mind, but its very foundation, from which it draws energy for its continued existence. The psychic is greater in scope than the ego, and among the psychic realities of the unconscious, man encounters forces which far transcend his personality. Consequently, it is necessary to come to terms with them, and whoever omits to do so falls a

[47] *WS*, p. 224.

victim to the perils of the soul. Jung has based his psychotherapeutic practice on the necessary fact that many people today feel themselves inwardly impelled to make this encounter. He has found out a great many things about unconscious psychic life and is of the opinion that much more is still to be discovered. To give but one example, he thinks that occult phenomena may prove to be new points of departure for discoveries in the field of the unconscious. Flournoy, of Genèva, in his examination of mediums, has put forward the hypothesis that under certain conditions psychic contents may be conjured out of the unconscious and appear in a manner that seems to us to border on the miraculous. Jung, too, devoted his first treatise to problems belonging to parapsychology; and in his later works he has not dropped the conjecture that this field may hold discoveries of the greatest interest to the psychology of the unconscious. He regards artistic symbolism, religion and mythology, alchemy and astrology as psychological documents which all have clues to offer to the zealous inquirer.

To conclude this summary, we shall list a few other concepts from Jungian psychology which we have either touched on or to which we shall have to return later.

Psychic contents that fall into the unconscious are as a result no longer bound up with the ego-function. They can start leading a life of their own in the unconscious and influence the conscious mind from there. Jung calls these *autonomous complexes;* they are active in the phenomena of neurosis, influencing and disturbing the ego. Disturbances of the conscious mind for which there is no sufficient reason in consciousness itself come from such autonomous complexes. They function most obviously in occult phenomena such as automatic writing. In all these cases we have to do with a nuclear element compounded of two things: an experience originating in the individual's surroundings, and a disposition of character. Round this element a number of associations crystallize, since psychic contents are very much "feeling-toned." Mostly the complexes are projected—unconsciously carried over into the surroundings. A historically famous instance of projection of an autonomous complex is witch-hunting. Jung was able to point out the workings of such complexes in his experiments with association. Autonomous complexes can be so constituted as to act like a second ego. The following function-complexes are particularly important:

a) The *shadow*. Not all our psychic functions and potentialities are equally developed; some are more differentiated than others, which are still in the crude state, so to speak. In his dealings with life a man makes use primarily of the faculties that are well developed in him; the rest fall into the unconscious, where they are not wholly lost but lead a shadow-existence. From there they ultimately give rise to man's "shadow": the complex of his inferior qualities. The shadow is a double which has many of the individual's qualities, but in reverse. His experience of the shadow sometimes intensifies into a vision of his "double," but as a rule the shadow is projected. We reproach others with, and attribute to them, the very things we have in ourselves and believe we have happily mastered. The religious believer, for instance, sees in other people all the possible doubts he has in himself. Every nation attributes to other nations what is really its own shadow.

b) Next the *persona*. By this Jung means the function that everybody develops in his dealings with the surrounding world. In necessarily adapting ourselves to reality, we present ourselves not as we really are, but, to put it bluntly, we play a part. As a rule this rôle is built up of a careful selection of our well-developed faculties plus their adaptation to the demands of the world. The persona would have us be not human beings with their own inherent contradictions but doctors, teachers, parsons, superiors, etc., ideal and perfect. Necessity demands that we adapt ourselves to reality; we cannot pass ourselves off as we would like to. We have to be fair to the wishes and demands of our fellows, because ultimately we need them. But we forget that we are playing a part and that our own personality is both smaller and greater than what we want to present to the world at large. One can thus say that the persona is the function through which we come to terms with our surroundings. It turns into an autonomous complex when a man ceases to bear in mind that his personality is not identical with it and that the persona is, as it were, the cloak for his ego. Then the persona either stifles his personality and the man becomes a psychic husk that is nothing more than the rôle he plays, or—a healthier but more painful proceeding—the tension between persona and personality leads to psychic suffering, sometimes verging on a neurosis, which can be resolved only by coming to terms with the persona and the counter-self, the shadow.

c) The third autonomous function is the *anima* or *animus*. The persona is the function whose business it is to come to terms with the outer world. Anima and animus do the same for the inner world. This function has a character that contradicts the individual's nature. Everybody has male and female ancestors. Consequently we each have, thanks to heredity, contra-sexual traits in ourselves: the man those of the woman, the woman those of the man. Adaptation to the world naturally requires the development of the traits corresponding to one's own sex. The others fall into the unconscious, but reappear in the function that establishes relations with the inner world. Therefore Jung calls this function the *anima* in men and the *animus* in women. Here too the unconscious displays its compensatory attitude by adding feminine traits to the man's consciousness and masculine to the woman's. The anima's nature is protean, uncanny. It manifests itself in a man's incalculable and obstinate moods, while the animus does so in a woman's equally obstinate, irritating, and ungrounded opinions. These functions, particularly the anima, are well suited to projection. Many men can tell even what their soul-image looks like, and this can often guide a man in his choice of a love-partner, for he may seek the anima in a real woman.

Here we will leave this field of Jungian psychology. By no means all the views put forward enjoy general recognition. For many people the whole thing is still too new and unknown for them to accept the whole of Jung's thought. Sometimes one really does get the impression that one is entering virgin territory where the explorer has to forge toilsomely ahead, feeling his way. For all that, the material Jung presents is extremely impressive. What does enjoy fairly widespread recognition, however, is Jung's view of the *psychological attitudes and types*, which we give herewith; and his distinction between introversion and extraversion. These too we give for the sake of completeness.

By *introversion* Jung means an inturning of interest resulting in a negative relation of subject to object. The subject's interest does not move towards the object but turns back to the subject. The introvert thinks, feels, and acts in a way which clearly shows that the subject is of prime interest, the object being allowed but a secondary

E

value. Introversion is active when the subject wants somehow to shut himself off from the object; passive, when he is incapable of restoring to the object the libido streaming back from it. If introversion is habitual Jung speaks of an introverted type.[48]

Extraversion is the direct opposite of introversion. "Extraversion means the outward-turning of libido. By this I mean an open relation of subject to object in the sense of a positive movement of subjective interest towards the object. A man in the extraverted state thinks, feels, and acts in relationship to the object and does so in a direct and clearly perceptible fashion, so that there can be no doubt of his positive attitude to the object. Extraversion is thus a sort of transportation of interest from subject to object. . . . In the extraverted state there is a strong, though not exclusive, determinism by the object. We can speak of active extraversion when the extraversion is deliberately willed; of passive extraversion when it is compelled by the object—that is to say, when the object attracts the subject's interest of its own accord, sometimes even against his will." [49] In the case of habitual extraversion Jung speaks of an extraverted type.

A distinction is therefore to be made between attitude and type. Under certain conditions a man may oscillate between the extraverted and the introverted attitude. Ultimately both attitudes are needful, because everybody has an inner world but lives in the outer world at the same time. Hence we all have both attitudes at our disposal, and only when one of them becomes habitual can we speak of a type. The reason why they produce a type is probably connected with man's psychic structure. But the exact reasons for this are unknown in the present state of psychological knowledge.

[48] *PT*, p. 641.   [49] *Ibid.*, p. 624.

Since, however, we all have both attitudes at our disposal, the one that is not preferred does not disappear altogether. According to the law of *enantiodromia* (the changing of a thing into its opposite), the neglected attitude may, when a certain point in life has been reached, become of prime importance. This can lead to conversions that may be religious, though not necessarily so. But the neglected attitude is always present in the shadow, and thus acquires an inferior character. It begins functioning when the individual's unconscious is somehow touched. For instance, when a man develops extraversion as the primary attitude, its valuable qualities are worked out and result in the happiest possible relationship to the external world. But the introversion sinks back into the unconscious and makes itself felt from there in unpredictable moods, etc. Since, therefore, we all have both attitudes at bottom and, in certain circumstances, realize them, it is often not at all easy to tell which attitude is typical in individual cases. It is particularly hard to discover to which type one belongs oneself.

But the distinction between extravert and introvert failed to satisfy Jung as constituting a real typology, for each of these types comprises persons of so varied a nature that a thoroughly satisfactory over-all description is lacking. Jung therefore looked for further marks of distinction and found that there are four fundamental psychic functions, of which people develop one particularly well as the primary function, while the other three are less developed or not at all. For Jung the psychological function is "a certain form of psychic activity that remains constant in principle under varying circumstances. Regarded as energy, the function is a manifestation of the libido, which itself remains constant in principle under varying conditions, much as physical strength can be regarded as one manifestation of physical energy." [50] Jung distinguishes four fundamental psychic functions, two of which are rational—thinking and feeling—and two irrational—sensation and intuition.

As to why they should be four in number, Jung says: "I can give no *a priori* reason why I call these functions the four basic functions; I can only stress the fact that this view has formed itself in me in the course of years of experience. I distinguish these functions from one another because they cannot be related or reduced to one another. The thinking-principle, for instance, is absolutely different from the feeling-principle, and so on. I also make a capital distinction between these functions and fantasy-thinking, because to my mind fantasy-thinking is a peculiar form of activity that can show itself in all four basic functions. Will seems to me to be an altogether secondary psychic phenomenon, likewise attention." [51]

For the sake of fuller understanding, it may be necessary to add Jung's definition of the rational and the irrational: "The rational is the reasonable, that which accords with reason. I conceive reason to be an attitude whose principle it is to mould thinking, feeling, and acting in accordance with objective values. Objective values are established by man's normal experience of external facts on the one hand, and of internal psychological ones on the other.... The rational attitude which allows us to assert objective values as valid at all is not, however, the work of the individual subject but of human history. Most objective values—and hence reason also—are solidly built complexes of ideas handed down to us from of old; their organization is the work of countless centuries operating with the same inevitability with which the na-

[50] *PT*, p. 628.   [51] *Ibid.*, p. 629.

ture of the living organism reacts to the normal and constantly repeated conditions of the surrounding world and builds up the functional complexes that correspond to them, e.g. the eye corresponding perfectly to the nature of light. ... Accordingly, human reason is the expression of man's adaptation to what is normally there, and this is deposited in complexes of ideas which, organizing themselves step by step, constitute objective values. The laws of reason are thus the laws which characterize and regulate the adapted attitude, the—on an average—'right' attitude. ... Thinking and feeling are rational functions in so far as they are decisively influenced by the element of reflection. They function at their best when they are in the fullest possible accord with the laws of reason." [52] The irrational is not the unreasonable but what is outside reason, namely that which cannot be grounded in reason —for instance, chance or the elementary facts of life. The rational functions are directed, the irrational not. Hence sensation and intuition function at their best not in explaining things but in the absolute perception of what is happening.

Jung describes the individual functions as follows:

Thinking brings ideas into an abstract pattern in accordance with their own laws. It is an apperceptive activity and can be active (volition) or passive (experience). The former is directed—intellectual thinking; it subjects ideas to deliberate judgement. The latter is undirected thinking, is intuitive, and arranges ideas by standards that are not conscious.

Feeling occurs between the ego and a given content and establishes its value in the sense of either accepting or rejecting it. When it occurs apart from the conscious content of the moment, it is mood. Feeling is a kind of

[52] *Ibid.*, pp. 658 *et seq.*

judgement, but not in the sense of establishing some connexion or other, rather with a view to acceptance or rejection. Ultimately it is the apperception of value.

Intuition transmits perceptions in an unconscious way. Both external and internal objects are apprehended by it. Intuition presents us with complete and finished contents, though we are not clear as to how they came into being. Jung distinguishes concrete and abstract intuition. The former intuits the possibility of things, the latter intuits ideal connexions.

Sensation transmits the physical stimuli of the sense-organs. It is sense-perception in the widest meaning of that word. It re-presents facts, also physiological impulses, but is not identical with them, since it is merely a perceptive function. Concrete sensation is always mixed with one of the other elementary functions—for instance, feeling. Abstract sensation is pure and the peculiar property of the artist.

These four functions are fundamental to everybody. One of them is given preference and dominates as the primary function. But the others are also there. Less energy is supplied to them and thus they belong in part to the unconscious. At the same time, these other three are not all equally developed: one of them is supplied with enough energy to be clearly detectable as a secondary function alongside the primary function. The third is likewise supplied with energy; only the fourth is completely neglected and allowed to fall entirely into the unconscious. We have to do, then, with the same process that we described as regards a man's attitude: one potentiality is developed and refined, while the others, though also latently there, are not realized. Consequently they fall to the shadow. When a man changes his attitude in a "conversion," a corresponding change occurs in the functions: the one that had hitherto been primary may be replaced by another.

Since, however, everybody normally holds fast to his primary function, this also gives rise to a type. Thus, there are thinking-types, feeling-types, intuition-types, and sensation-types. And since each of these four function-types can be either extraverted or introverted, Jung arrives at eight types in all: the extraverted thinking-type, the introverted thinking-type, the extraverted feeling-type, the introverted feeling-type, etc. In this way he has devised a differential typology as it emerged from his medical practice.

We believe we have now described the elements of Jungian psychology as far as it is pertinent to our purpose. But over and above all the individual details we must always bear in mind Jung's basic views, which can be summed up roughly as follows:

1. Man takes his stand in an inner as well as an outer world, both of which are significant and fateful for him.

2. All experience passes through the psyche. Experience of our environment can be apprehended only in pictures that the environment releases in us. All experience, that of extraneous life included, is always bound up with self-experience.

3. Everything to do with the soul is real, i.e. actual; and the psychic, even though it may have no counterpart in the external world, acts and is therefore true.

4. Soul is life and is only experienceable as life.

5. Soul is greater than the ego and consciousness; this is only a little island in the ocean of psychic reality, in which the individual personality is contained as the physical individual is contained in the physical world.

THE PSYCHIC BASES OF RELIGION

T̶URNING now to our theme, the psychology of religion as found in Jung, we shall deal first of all with the why and wherefore of religious experiences. We shall try to answer the question regarding the psychic sphere in which religious experience occurs and the psychic mechanisms whose function it involves.

For a long time it was almost a dogma with many people, theologians and others, that the sublime nature of religious experience exalted it above all other psychic processes. They denied altogether that religious experience was accessible to psychology. This standpoint has still not been abandoned by many theologians even today. They categorically refuse to acknowledge that the psyche has anything to do with religion, revelation, and faith. These things, they say, are miles away from man's psychic life and lie on a totally different plane. Such a standpoint is, in a sense, consistent and extremely simple. It can also be associated very easily with the view that man is tainted with original sin and an utterly wretched creature in consequence, whom the metaphysician can accuse of all sorts of defects and who can be so moulded by the pastor of souls that he will eventually believe the message of salvation announced to him—in other words, acknowledge it as right if only he sacrifices his reason. Unfortunately, the last three hundred years have shown more and more that this doctrine, even theologically, is not without its difficulties. It and its consequences proved to be in conflict with other branches of knowledge which could also claim a certain plausibility; and finally notice had to be taken of the fact that, for many people, this appeal to all their feelings of inferiority was unable, despite the announcement of divine salvation following closely on its heels, despite the promise of rescue from the welter of their sins, really to help them in their troubles. So people came to give up the view that religion had nothing to do with man's soul, together with the kindred view of the "natural" man. They did not, however, go to the point of confounding soul and religion in one common ruin, but availed themselves of another possibility of safeguarding the sublime nature of religion, namely by reserving a special field for it which was piously fenced off from that of instinct and ordinary, everyday impulses and thoughts. Only the most transcendent feelings and the most elevated thoughts and purely spiritual impulses were connected with religion. Everything else was mere psychic life, which was naturally not allowed to have anything to do with religious experience. This attitude is about as legitimate as thinking that Raphael or Rembrandt must have painted with far more precious and dignified oils than the ordinary painter whose fame has not penetrated beyond his local habitat.

Many people—scientists or thinkers of no particular academic profession—had long known that the facts were otherwise. But it needed the scandal of a Freud to bruit these ideas abroad on any large scale. When Freud came and brought religion into connexion, indeed intimate relation, with the ordinary impulses of the human psyche and even with instinctual life, great was the scandalization and horror of many people on account of such godlessness, and equally natural the uproar it occasioned. They repudiated Freud's views vehemently and unequivocally, but Freud had accomplished one thing: people began to busy themselves with the question whether it might not in the end be that religion and the soul were closer together than they had seemed heretofore. That Freud intentionally and in many cases quite justifiably questioned the alleged sublimity of certain fields of human life was of the nature of his work, and it is to his credit to have done so. Even religion had something to thank him for, since he brought it nearer to life.

There has probably never been any doubt for Jung that religion is either a psychic occurrence and thus intimately connected with the total structure of the soul, or is nothing at all. He does not hesitate to regard religious experience as accessible to psychology, and he makes no fundamental distinction between religious processes and other psychic happenings. With complete impartiality he sets them side by side in his writings, and tries to establish the inner connexion between them, without worrying whether the loftiness of religion, which seems to lie so close to the hearts of some people, is thereby preserved. You get the impression from his literary work that the question as to the rightness of this attitude has never even occurred to him, and that he became conscious of it only with the reception accorded to his little book *Psychology and Religion*. The discussions aroused at the time showed him that many theological readers were irritated by his impartiality in bringing religion and psychology together. It was only in his Introduction to *Psychology and Alchemy* that he tried to enter into considerations of that kind.

One great innovation strikes you at once in Jung's psychological researches into religion: that is the significance he attaches to the unconscious in religious life. As we have seen in our sketch of Jung's views, he holds that the unconscious is just as important as the conscious mind. This is unconditionally true of religion also. Jung is very much concerned with the psychic wholeness of man. We shall see later on that this wholeness has a strong bearing on religion, and that religion in its turn has certain definite functions in the integration of personality. Hence, from this point of view as well, Jung had to take thorough cognizance of the unconscious functions in religious experience. But that in itself was not a motive for stressing the actuality of the unconscious so much as Jung's ultimate opinion that the unconscious is the seat of the religious function.[1] This implies a reversal of many traditional views, for until now religion was essentially bound up with mind and spirit. People knew from religious history that other religions did exist; but those that were not "spiritual" religions were called "nature-religions" and regarded as a phase that humanity would outgrow. When Freud put religion and the unconscious side by side, there were no dire results. For Freud himself wanted the destruction of religion, and those who still valued it, despite Freud, either repudiated his ideas *in toto* as anti-religious propaganda, or acknowledged the influence of the unconscious in the pathological forms of religion at most, not in "real" religion. Only William James had foreseen the possibility of unconscious processes influencing religious experience, namely in conversion. Jung, on the other hand, asserted that religion affected the whole man and his entire psychic personality, hence also the unconscious; and further, that the essential processes of religious life took place not in the spirit, not in the feelings or the reason, but in the unconscious.

Thus Jung traces back to the unconscious the "inner

[1] *PR*, p. 11.

voice" so important to every religious person, the voice of revelation. "Revelation," says Jung, "is an opening of the depths of the human soul, a 'laying bare,' a psychological mode pure and simple, which says nothing about what *else* it could be. That lies outside the bounds of science."[2] What is at the bottom of these processes Jung refuses to conjecture; but this much is certain for him, that what we experience as revelation comes from the unconscious. Lest we should misunderstand Jung at the outset, we must at once add by way of a reminder that "unconscious" does not mean "deriving from *one's own* personality," since psychic reality exists over and above personality and ego. What we are dealing with, therefore, is a psychic realm far removed from all human volition and influence. Let us remember, however, Jung's view that the unconscious can give rise to highly meaningful events—meaningful for man's personality as a whole. This is also true in the matter of religion. Jung has no qualms about citing the Old Testament prophets as witnesses to his view that the unconscious has a revelatory significance, since they regarded dreams as revelations. "The remarkable fact that the dream is a divine voice and message on the one hand and an unending source of trouble on the other does not disturb the primitive mind. We find perceptible traces of this primitive fact in the psychology of the Hebrew prophets. Often they hesitated to harken to the voice. And admittedly it was a hard thing for a pious man like Hosea to marry a harlot in order to obey the Lord's command."[3] Jung then goes on to say that the Church has limited the significance of dreams for religious life, because a too zealous observation of the voice of the unconscious imperils the observance of dogma. But the Church has always ac-

² *Ibid.*, p. 133.   ³ *Ibid.*, p. 34.

knowledged the possibility that dreams could contain genuine revelations. "Thus the change of mental attitude that has occurred in the last few centuries is, from this point of view at least, not wholly unwelcome to the Church, seeing that the earlier introspective attitude that favoured a serious concern with dreams and inner experiences was thereby effectively discouraged."[4] Hence, according to Jung, it is only in recent centuries that the voice of the unconscious has ceased to be recognized as significant for religion. His own views he regards as a sort of insight that had been common property long before psychology became a science. Inner experiences, dreams included, were always part of the religious man's make-up.

Jung would have the unconscious play a special part in religious conversions. The American school of religious psychology early began to devote considerable study to this problem, though the studies were extensive rather than intensive. William James was the first to go into conversion, not only to attack it with questionnaires and all the paraphernalia proper to the religious psychology of the time, but also to interpret it. This led him, as said above, to the idea that the unconscious was also at work. James stopped at this conjecture, as he was not equipped to interpret the workings of the unconscious in any profounder sense. Jungian psychology is in a position to penetrate deeper.

The basis of conversion is the ability of the unconscious to activate itself spontaneously whenever consciousness make this necessary. That is, when the conscious mind favours and fosters an attitude in a one-sided manner that fails to satisfy the needs of the total personality, an untenable psychic situation is gradually

4 *Ibid.,* p. 35.

brought about. If the conscious mind is unable to correct its one-sidedness, the compensatory activity of the unconscious begins to function. The unconscious sets about preparing a new attitude which is then released at a certain moment and transforms consciousness. The individual experiences this as a complete transformation of personality, all the more startling since it all happens in a moment. If he wanted consciously to change his attitude—which sometimes is the case—he would need far more time. The old attitude disappears from consciousness but is not wholly dissolved; it remains latent in the unconscious and goes on exerting a certain influence from there. The whole process follows the law of enantiodromia, according to which every attitude that implies one-sidedness calls up in the unconscious a compensatory attitude.[5] The interesting thing about Jung's explanation of conversion is that the first attitude does not disappear altogether but remains latent. It can make itself felt in various bodily disturbances—which is how Jung explains the epileptic fits of the apostle Paul. What Jung has to say in his memorial address on Richard Wilhelm is relevant here. Wilhelm, working as a Christian missionary in China, acquainted himself with the wisdom of the Chinese, their philosophy and religion, and eventually became their proselyte in Europe. But, although in his thought he turned strongly to the East, his religious ties with Europe and Christianity were unbroken; and Jung sees in this pull between his latent Christianity and his conscious orientation to the spirit of China the final cause of Wilhem's sufferings and early death [6]

Jung shows that sudden conversions do not in fact happen, as had long been supposed. The new attitude has been prepared in the unconscious; the only surprising thing is

[5] *PT*, p. 621.   [6] *The Secret of the Golden Flower*, p. 77 et seq.

the suddenness of its emergence into consciousness. But it would be possible for an observer who could see into the soul and above all into dreams and fantasies to note the imminent change of personality long beforehand. At the same time, Jung shows that the significance of the conversion should not be overestimated. The suddenness of the event makes it very portentous for the individual concerned, so that he is inclined to set a high value on it. But if converts think that they have experienced a transformation of their whole personality, that is only a subjective delusion. All that has happened is a change of attitude, not of the whole man. And as Jung points out, the old Adam—the attitude that has been dropped—is still latent and can operate from the unconscious. The new attitude born of conversion may very well be one-sided in its turn; it has come into being by way of compensation to another one-sidedness, and this says nothing about the personality, the totality of the inner man, itself being enlarged. One has only to remember the one-sidedness of, say, St. Augustine after his conversion and how in many respects he went from one extreme to the other, to see that Jung is right on this point. At all events, there is still the possibility of yet other changes that may be psychically more important than conversion, though in many circles this is looked upon as the culmination of religious experience. It only remains to remark that the history of Christianity from Paul to the present offers a wealth of material for interpretation in terms of the law of enantiodromia.

The psychology of the unconscious also offers an interpretation of various other factors in religious life—above all, of myth. In this respect Jung's depth-psychology has thrown up many new points of view. Theological research into religion has always regarded mythology as one of the most difficult problems and still does so, unless it prefers to pass the whole thing over in silence. Two problems keep cropping up again and again: firstly, what is the real meaning and value of myths? and secondly, why are similar themes and motifs to be met with all over the world in mythology? To begin with the second problem: Students of comparative religion have always assumed so far that the various religions and religious cultures mutually influenced one another. The best known if not the only theory proposed in answer to this question is pan-Babylonism, which traces the affinity of motifs in the myths of various peoples to the old Babylonian religion. It is tempting, when faced with such mythological correspondences, to think of the myths migrating from country to country and even across the seas. But in due course science had to admit that things did not happen like that, since it is not so easy for a people really to be influenced in its religion by that of a foreign people, which one would have to assume according to this theory. Very often nothing of the sort could be proved.

The question as to the nature of myth proved even more difficult. The most plausible explanation was that myths, for one thing, contained certain ancestral memories of prehistoric events and, for another, were a primitive explanation of nature. The enlightened nineteenth century, so proud of its newly created science and the techniques associated with it, was very prone to interpretations of this sort. Unfortunately, however, these had the disadvantage of not answering all the questions satisfactorily. It is understandable that a primitive Negro tribe should explain natural happenings like this, but not the Greeks, who were intelligent enough to have evolved a natural science of their own. But myth still played an overwhelming part in the life of the Greeks, as Homer and the classical Greek theatre show. If the Greeks let mythological figures take the stage at the height of their culture, this fact is not to be explained as primitive science or inadequate knowledge of history. There is more to it than that.

Further, any concern with mythology always harbours a particularly painful problem for the theologian—namely, the relationship between Christianity and myth. The Christian theologian will obviously say in advance that no such relationship exists. The Christian religion, he holds, is far above every mythology. What it offers is revelation, and to associate revelation with mythology is both presumptuous and fallacious, if not downright blasphemous. We can wilfully ignore this problem or execrate the godlessness and neo-paganism of those who have raised it, but it is still there. We have only to study Albert Schweitzer's history of research into the life of Jesus to see that even the examination of the historical figure of Jesus raises the question of whether Christianity has assimilated its meed of mythological material. D. F. Strauss sets the figure of Jesus alongside the figures of mythology and establishes that correspondences exist. Those who contest the historicity of Jesus interpret all the reports of the evangelists in terms of mythology. Schweitzer, explaining Jesus' *Weltanschauung* in the light of late Judaic apocalypticism, also goes back to mythological motifs. Controversy as to the rights and wrongs of Schweitzer's thesis still rages today. He has not met with general recognition, but it can comfortably be stated that no historical interpretation of Jesus has been brought forward to date that can lay claim to greater scientific probability. If one refuses to acknowledge this, one must without exception reject in principle all scientific and

68

historical researches into the figure of Jesus. At any rate, the state of our knowledge at present confirms that mythological motifs do in fact appear in the evangelical writings on Jesus, and that Jesus himself lived in a mental atmosphere that was saturated with mythological elements. The same thing is true of Paul, the New Testament in general, and the nascent Christian Church. Here, too, we find mythological motifs everywhere. But are all these so many primitive attempts to explain things? The idea can scarcely be supported.

Jung goes into all three questions on the following fundamental principle: myth is the projection of man's unconscious, and the collective unconscious at that. What we find pictured in the myths of the various peoples and religions is not the imperfect image of certain portions of the external world, but the projection of the unconscious inner world. Lest any misunderstanding should arise we should really say: myth is the projection of that part of psychic reality which is accessible to us in the collective unconscious. Myth rests on inner experience, though not on the ego's experience; it rests rather on the experience of powers, processes, and happenings that lie beyond one's own ego. Myth is the graphic representation of man's experience of psychic forces.[7]

With this the first question is answered for Jung. The collective unconscious re-presents the memories not only of the individual man but of all mankind. In it are contained the instincts and their psychic analogues—the archetypes. Since the latter rest on age-old experience, they contain fragments of earlier stages of development. Just as the structure of the body contains vestiges of evolutionary periods now outgrown, so it is with the collective

[7] *SPG*, p. 166.

unconscious; and accordingly it exhibits features that correspond to one another in all peoples and races. Because it has remained the same in the different races of mankind and in different periods, it is understandable that correspondences should occur in the field of myth. In this we see a correspondence in the structure of the psyche itself, hence there is no need to explain this correspondence by the influence of the various peoples on one another or by the carrying over of myth-motifs. As the myth is a projection of psychic occurrences in the collective unconscious, a correspondence will naturally result among peoples of different races, cultures, and periods. Jung has in fact shown that myth-motifs are still present in modern civilized man. He first noted this astonishing fact with the mentally deranged; and then careful examination of the dreams of mentally healthy persons proved that they too may, under certain conditions, produce mythological processes and events in their dreams. So that the civilized man of today still has myth, or the basis of it—the experiences of the collective unconscious—at work in himself, but his attention is riveted on the external world to such an extent that he scarcely notices it and therefore keeps it unconscious. Only in dreams and fantasies does it come to light.

The second question is also answered for Jung, concerning the meaning and value of myths. The idea that myths are an imperfect explanation of natural phenomena or an inadequate way of expressing memorable historical events does not hold water. It is obvious that motifs of this kind are also present in later periods, but they are never the main thing. Myth is primarily the experience and expression of what happens in the soul. For those to whom myth is a living thing, it conveys a meaning as shattering as that which is given to us in the experience of revelation.[8] It is experienced as such by the primitive mind. Myth is never a matter of caprice, of the desire for amusement, or of make-believe with an illusory world that masks the grimness of reality—as, for instance, in the case of factory-girls today with the help of the cinema; it is always a way of expressing profoundly moving experiences. It voices the aspirations, the struggles, and also the horror and terror that are inevitably bound up with human existence. It conceals experiences that probably do not fall short, in intensity, of those of the insane. For whoever lives in the world of myth experiences the might of the unconscious, the same forces which mental sufferers also have to do with—the same forces, too, which afflict mankind with mass-possession in times of historical crisis such as the French Revolution or, indeed, today. One has only to bear classical drama in mind to realize the fearful psychic reality that lies behind it. Myth has no rational meaning in the sense that man is aiming at something or wants to reach something. But there is some terrific experience at the back of it which man wants to formulate somehow and must express, just as the artist is compelled to give his experiences plastic shape. He is seized by suprapersonal powers and portrays them in his myths in a way that all who have ever experienced them can understand.

In what is his key work in this respect—the *Psychology of the Unconscious*—Jung elaborates the idea that in myth we have, *inter alia*, self-portraits of the movements of the libido. Thus the sun, the snake, fire, the horse are its symbols. Further, myths contain pictures of the archetypes. In the above book he cites the tree and the *temenos* as representations of the mother-archetype. The desire

[8] Jung-Kerényi: *Introduction to a Science of Mythology*, London, 1950, p. 102

71

to go back to the mother is the desire to go back to the mother's womb. This theme myths represent as the act of being *devoured*. The tree is likewise a mother-symbol. The "tree of the dead," as the coffin is called in many parts of the world, is a mother-symbol, too; and entombment is the return to the mother. So is the hanging on a tree, or crucifixion; for the tree-image, hence the mother-symbol, may be concealed in the cross. This return to the mother, to the origin, is supposed to effect an increase and renewal of libido. It is the pre-condition of rebirth and transformation. Similarly, mythological images of the course of the sun are expressions of movements of the libido. If they speak of the sun's nocturnal journey, it means a regression of libido, while the sun's journey across the heavens means progression. Together they may be taken as expressing Goethe's "systole and diastole"—a rhythm that is certainly known to man. When he experiences a change, or when something new is born in him, it is represented by the symbol of the birth of a god. Inner formations of this kind are constantly being threatened by various psychic impulses, and this threat is symbolized by the enemies who always menace the birth of a religious founder—e.g. the massacre of the innocents.

Here we have reached Jung's answer to the third problem, the question of the relation of Christianity to myth. Jung takes it as a matter of course that myths are also at work in Christianity, and, as regards his view that the collective unconscious is universal in range, this could hardly be otherwise. In the book above mentioned, he gives many examples of how myth-motifs are present in Christian art, doctrine, and even the New Testament. For instance, the dragon that threatens to devour the hero about to be born is a mythological image. It means the libido that is trying to get back to the mother and is hostile to the birth of a new personality. This dragon-motif also crops up in connection with Jesus, as the antichrist. Jung mentions a cup used at the Last Supper with a dragon on it.[9] Christianity employs numerous other libido-symbols—fire, for instance; witness the apocryphal saying of our Lord: "He who is near to me is near to the fire." The fish, well known to have been used very frequently in primitive Christianity, is a libido-symbol in other religions as well. Generally it is explained as a pictogram of the Greek word ICHTHYS, which comprises the initial letters of Jesus' title: *Jesu Christos Theou Yios Soter*—Jesus Christ Son of God Redeemer. Jung thinks it more probable that the libido-symbol is the real motif of this sign. Ultimately, the fish is a phallic symbol and hence a libido-symbol. Jung also shows that there are pictures of Jesus in which he is represented as an androgyne, as is the case with other redeemer-gods. Water too can be a libido-symbol, though the Christian Church knew it as baptismal water. Further, the mother-archetype has a great part to play. It appears in the guise of the city, e.g. the Heavenly Jerusalem in the Revelation of St. John. The altar and the font may likewise be mother-symbols, representing the womb. In the Crucifixion between the thieves we have the Dioscuri-motif, which symbolizes the mortal and the immortal. The temptations of Jesus during the forty days in the wilderness contain a spiritualized version of the fight with the dragon, a theme clearly developed in Mithraism. Jung also sees in Christianity parallels to the cults of Ceres and Dionysus, for which he cites the vine-motif in the Johannine sayings. A very widespread mythological theme shows the hero's father as an arrowsmith or carpenter, meaning that he is the begetter of excellent sons. Arrows are libido-symbols. In mythology we often

[9] *WSL*, p. 402.

come across two mothers and the allied idea of a second birth. This can be represented as a re-finding (the twelve-year-old Jesus in the temple). The two-mother-motif has had its effect on Christian dogma, in that the Holy Ghost is sometimes interpreted as feminine. Lastly, primitive mythology has the image of the solar phallus. In Christian art this theme appears in certain representations of the Pentecostal fire, also in those of the Immaculate Conception. These examples may suffice to show that Jung sees the processes of the collective unconscious portrayed as mythological images which occur not only in the religions outside Christianity but within the fold of the Christian Church, in its worship, dogma, art, and legends. It must be remarked here that in his investigations of Christianity Jung has taken account not only of the established churches and generally accepted doctrines, but also of all the possible sects and esoteric traditions, particularly the Gnostic doctrines. The reason for this will become apparent in the sequel.

In dealing with certain other factors in religion, Jung also points to the psychological background. For instance, he traces the belief in a diversity of gods to autonomous complexes. The psyche sometimes splits off certain portions from the ego. This is mostly the case when the ego-function is not very strongly developed; and in earlier periods of recorded history—not by any means only in the primitive religions and cultures—man clearly had a weaker ego as the focus of personality than he has today. His soul was, so to speak, less centralized, and the fissiparous tendency showed itself also in his views of deity. He did not know a uniform God who creates and controls everything, but a multiplicity of gods corresponding to the structure of his own psyche.[10] Like split-off complexes,

[10] *The Secret of the Golden Flower*, p. 109.

the many individual gods in such a pantheon each lead a life of their own. Whether a people will profess a polytheistic or a monotheistic religion, therefore, depends on psychological factors, since belief in one God or several gods corresponds to a given psychic situation. The belief, too, that the individual has a diversity of souls and the belief in the existence of spirits are likewise psychologically conditioned. When a people believes in a man's having more than one soul, what we are dealing with is a multiplicity of relatively autonomous complexes all belonging to the personal unconscious. That is why the loss of a soul is regarded as harmful: all the souls must remain in the vicinity of the ego. Spirits likewise are autonomous complexes, but of the collective unconscious, and thus supra-personal in nature. Since they have no direct connexion with the ego, they are projected—in contrast to the souls which a man feels as residing in himself. As complexes of the collective unconscious, spirits cannot and must not be bound to the ego, otherwise they would overpower it, and possession would result. For Jung it is a confirmation of the difference between the personal and collective unconscious that the primitive view of things distinguishes two causes of illness: namely, possession by spirits or loss of a soul. As complexes of the personal unconscious, souls must remain bound to the ego; their loss is injurious to personality, whereas spirits, being functions of the collective unconscious, are projected and are not permitted to impinge too closely on personality lest they overwhelm it.[11]

Jung also traces the belief in immortality to certain aspects of the soul. "The quality of immortality," he says, "may well owe its origin . . . to the specifically historical

[11] *UES*, p. 213.

aspect of the soul. . . . When the Buddhists say that progressive perfection through concentration leads to the remembrance of former incarnations, they are probably referring to the same psychological fact, the only difference being that they ascribe the historical factor not to the soul but to the self. It is quite in keeping with the completely extraverted mentality of the West up to now that by feeling (and tradition) we should ascribe immortality to a soul which we distinguish more or less from the ego, and which is also distinguished from it by its feminine qualities. It would be quite logical if now, by a deepening of the hitherto neglected introvert frame of mind, a change were brought about akin to the Eastern, and the quality of immortality transferred itself from the ambiguous figure of the soul (anima) to the self. It is essentially our over-estimation of external material objects that constellates an immortal spiritual figure within us, naturally for the purpose of compensation and self-adjustment. At bottom the historical factor attaches not merely to the feminine archetype but to all archetypes whatever—that is to say, to all hereditary units, mental as well as physical. Our life is what it has been for countless ages. In our sense of the word it is not a transitory thing, for the same physiological and psychological processes that have belonged to man for hundreds and thousands of years still persist and give us in our inmost hearts the deepest possible premonition of the 'eternal' continuity of all that lives. Our self, however, in the sense of something that embraces the whole living system, does not merely contain the total deposit of all the life that has ever been lived; it is also a point of departure, the pregnant womb of all future life, foreknowledge of which is given to our inmost selves as clearly as is life's historical aspect. The idea of immortality arises quite legitimately from this psychological background." [12] Hence, as these interesting statements show, the idea of immortality is grounded in the psyche; and Jung points out that the form in which the Christianity of the West knows it— the immortality of the *soul*—is determined by the intrinsically extravert attitude of mind that "constellates" the soul-image. In this respect, dogma as well is based on that psychic constellation.

Jung even proves this in the case of the doctrine of the Trinity. He has gone very deeply into the psychological background, chiefly in connexion with his studies on alchemy. He is of the opinion that the Trinity is not just a mystification devised by the human mind, but that behind it there lie revelations of the depths of the human soul. He gives full assent to what the Catholic writer Koepgen says in his book *Die Gnosis des Christentums*: "Thus the Trinity is a revelation not only of God but at the same time of man." [18] What may ultimately lie at the back of such religious forms is difficult to say, our knowledge of the structure of the human soul being what it is; but Jung is convinced that the Trinity contains pointers to psychic facts. That we should attribute a special significance to the numbers three and four is bound up with our whole psychic disposition. The theologian will take cognizance of such views only with the greatest misgiving. For all that, Jung finds himself in excellent company. No less an authority than St. Augustine himself, in his *De trinitate*, refers back to the soul in order to elucidate his teachings on the triune God. Had this theologian not felt that a certain relationship must exist between the soul and the doctrine of the Trinity he would hardly have seized on this thought. In recent

[12] *BZIU*, pp. 123 *et seq.*   [18] *PR*, p. 133.

times, Adolf Schlatter, the Protestant dogmatist of Tübingen, has likewise taken man as the starting-point for his teachings about God. Schlatter's "doctrine of faith"—he himself has been rated a Biblicist, but he has always gone his own, very often unique, way—sees that between experience of the self and intuition of God there are certain affinities that are crucial when it comes to expressing our experience of God. So that though Jung's ideas may be disconcerting for theology, they are not quite so alien as one might at first think.

The differences in human types also make themselves felt in the religious context. In his *Varieties of Religious Experience*, William James went into the same question. He possessed, of course, no thoroughgoing knowledge of human types and worked simply with the old doctrine of the four temperaments; but he managed to show that each man's religion is coloured according to his feelings. Jung, in his *Psychological Types*, has proved his thesis with a wealth of material drawn from the history of church and dogma. The speculations and flashes of insight it contains are so interesting that we shall cite a few of them. Thus, Jung proves beyond doubt that Tertullian was a typical introverted thinker. Origen, on the other hand, was essentially an extravert. In their religious development both men sacrificed their specific type as an offering to God. They knew it was necessary for man to sacrifice himself, and they each did so in such a way as to offer up the very qualities that were most highly developed in them. Tertullian sacrificed his intellect: he preached faith—the faith than can be won only by submitting to the irrational ("*credo, quia absurdum*"); and he acknowledged feeling to the degree that the thinker in him inevitably resisted it. This is why he finally went over to the Montanists—a sect that expected the end of the world at any moment and indulged in eschatological ecstasies. Origen, as an extravert, sacrificed the instinct which relates man most powerfully to his surroundings—sexuality: he castrated himself.[14]

Jung sees the opposition between the two types also working itself out in theological conflicts. We dispute because in the last resort we do not understand, in the things that concern us most deeply, that we belong to different psychological types. A psychological opposition of this kind is apparent, Jung thinks, in the fight over *homoousia* and *homoiousia;* in the fight between Ratramnus and Radbertus over the Communion, and in the tremendous battle about nominalism and realism that raged all through the Middle Ages. As is probably well known, the discussion hinged on whether ideas and concepts are only names, or are realities. The nominalist called them names only, thus displaying a typically extraverted attitude. The realist regarded ideas as realities and thus proved himself an introvert. According to Jung, the argument between Pelagius and Augustine also rests on a type-difference, since Pelagius was markedly extravert, Augustine introvert. Anselm's proof of the existence of God Jung regards as a characteristic piece of introverted thinking. Anselm taught that God is perfect, otherwise he would not be God. But it is essential to the perfection of a being that it should also exist. Therefore God, as perfect Being, must be. At the back of this argument there is a notion of the *efficacy* of ideas that is characteristic of the introvert but by no means so obvious to the extravert. Jung also thinks it possible to detect characteristic differences between introverts and extraverts in their way of apprehending God. The extravert is always inclined to think of God as

14 *PT*, pp. 22 *et seq.*

changing and evolving, while the introvert sees God as remaining the same. Finally, the conflict over the Communion between the reformers rests partly on the psychological differences between Luther and Zwingli. Luther was more an extravert, Zwingli introvert. Of course, other factors were involved, as we shall see later. But these brief indications show at all events that the psychological type is related to the manner in which a man experiences religion. We cannot go very far in our conclusions as yet, since Jung himself says that our present knowledge of psychological types is very imperfect. Many gaps remain to be filled in, and as regards the structure of the soul there are more questions than assured statements. But we can safely assert that the psychologist has successfully established certain relationships between the facts of religious life and the facts of psychic life.

At this point we must refer to one of the most important psychological manifestations of religion, namely the symbol. Jung comes to speak again and again of the symbol, and it can almost be said that Jung has rediscovered the symbol for many people, scientists included. In an age of rationalism and intellectualism the symbol has received scant attention and its significance has gone unappreciated. It was generally—not without deeper reasons—confused with allegory and the *sign* as ordinarily understood. Nor does modern Protestant theology in any of its branches pay much attention to it. In all foreign religions the symbol is of the highest significance. Only Protestantism has largely done away with it and regards it with suspicion, instantly scenting in all religious cults and rites and in all art within the precincts of the Church a papist tendency. But if Protestantism is right from its own point of view to refuse to rate the religious value of the symbol very high (later we shall come to the reason for this), it still should not overlook the fact that for many religious persons the symbol is *the* expression of faith and cannot be replaced by a better; and that only those who have found access of some kind to the symbol can have any idea of what religious experience really means to such persons. It is no small merit of modern psychology to have recognized the full value of the symbol.

"The symbol as I see it," says Jung, "is to be distinguished strictly from the mere sign. Symbolical and semiotic meanings are totally different things. In his book *Les Lois psychologiques du symbolisme*, Ferrero does not speak of symbols, but of signs. For instance, the old custom of handing over a sod of earth at the sale of a piece of land may vulgarly be described as 'symbolical,' but its nature is purely semiotic. The sod of earth is a sign or token for the bit of land as a whole. The winged wheel on the uniform of the railway official is not a symbol of the railway, but a sign that distinguishes the personnel of this railway. The symbol, on the other hand, always presupposes that the expression chosen is the best possible designation or formula for a relatively unknown fact which is still known, or required, to exist. ...Any view that explains the symbolical expression as an analogy or as an abbreviated description of a known fact is semiotic. But the view that explains the symbolical expression as the best possible formulation of a relatively unknown fact which cannot conceivably, therefore, be more clearly or characteristically represented, is symbolical. Again, a view that explains the symbolical expression as the intentional description, or rather circumscription, of a known fact is allegorical. To explain the cross as a 'symbol of divine love' is semiotic, since 'divine love' describes the fact to be expressed more tellingly and far better than a cross, which can have many other meanings. We are talking symbolically, however, when, over and above all thinkable explanations, we regard the cross as the expression for an as yet unknown and unintelligible fact of a mystical or transcendental—hence psychological—character, which can most fittingly be represented by a cross. As long as a symbol is alive it is expressive of a fact that could not be described better in any other way. The symbol is only alive so long as it is pregnant with meaning. But once it has given birth to its meaning, that is to say, once that expression is found which formulates the thing sought, expected, or guessed at, even better than the previous symbol did, then the symbol is dead, i.e. is only of historical significance. We can still speak of it as a symbol, but on the tacit understanding that we are speaking of it as it was *before* it had given birth to its better expression. The way in which Paul and the older mystics treat the symbol of the cross shows that it was a living symbol for them, something that expressed the inexpressible in a manner that could not be surpassed. All esoteric explanations kill the symbol, for esotericism develops better—often only supposedly better—expressions for it and thus reduces it to a merely conventional sign for relationships which are better and more completely understood elsewhere." [15] Thus, it depends on the person concerned and his whole psychological make-up whether a thing is symbolical for him or not. The same thing can be symbolical for one person and not for another, according to the state of psychic development of each.

Whether I take a thing as a symbol depends on whether I expect it to appear symbolical. "Whether

[15] *Ibid.*, pp. 674 *et seq.*

something is a symbol or not depends primarily on the attitude of the mind that observes it, the attitude of mind, for instance, which regards the thing given not merely as such but as an expression of the unknown. It is quite possible, therefore, for a man to produce a fact that has nothing symbolical about it to his way of thinking, but may be profoundly symbolical to another. The converse is also possible. There are, however, products whose symbolical character depends not merely on the attitude of the observing mind, but reveals itself quite spontaneously in the symbolical effect it has on the observer. Such products are so constituted that they would inevitably lack all meaning were they not invested with a symbolical one. A triangle enclosing an eye is, as a matter of fact, so essentially meaningless that the observer cannot possibly take it as a mere bit of chance foolery. A figure of this sort at once obtrudes itself as a symbol. This effect is strengthened either by the frequent and identical occurrence of the same figure, or else by the figure's being produced with particular care, which means that it is being used to express a particular value that has been superimposed on it. Symbols that do not work in the way just described are either dead, i.e. supplanted by a better formulation, or are products whose symbolical nature ultimately depends on the attitude of the observing mind. We can call the attitude that takes the thing given as a symbol, the 'symbolic attitude' for short." [16]

In many cases it is difficult to say whether a symbol is alive or not. We can appreciate a symbol in its historical significance and afterwards, feeling our way, try to understand what it means. This adaptation of feeling often attains a fairly high degree of living sympathy:

[16] *Ibid.*, p. 677.

we have only to think of the Romantic penchant for mediaeval symbols or our own tendency to appropriate symbols from the East. But the interest is more an aesthetic one, and when we come to ask ourselves what such symbols ultimately mean to us we soon reach the question of the genuineness of our religion and outlook —a very urgent if difficult problem today.

As to the psychological elements of the symbol, Jung says: "The living symbol is the formulation of an essentially unconscious component, and the more universal this component is the more universal is the effect of the symbol, since it will touch a chord in each of us. Since, on the one hand, the symbol is the best possible expression that the epoch in question has devised for the as yet unknown quantity, it must come from the most highly differentiated and complicated layer of the contemporary spiritual atmosphere. But since, on the other hand, the living symbol must, if it is to work at all, contain something that has affinities with a sizable group of human beings, it will inevitably comprise precisely what can be common to that group. Now this can never be anything very highly differentiated, nor the highest attainable, which only the few can reach and understand; it must be something still so primitive that none can have any doubt as to its omnipresence. Only when the symbol grasps this primitive factor and brings the expression of it to the highest pitch does it enjoy universal effect. Therein lies the tremendous and at the same time the saving power of a living social symbol." [17] Again: "The symbol is a structure of the utmost complexity, since data deriving from every psychic function have entered into its composition. Consequently, it is neither rational nor irrational in nature. It has a side that is agreeable to reason, but

[17] Ibid., p. 679.

also a side to which reason has no access, being composed not only of rational data but of the irrational data of pure inward and outward perception. The symbol is full of inklings and meanings and thus appeals to thought as well as to feeling; and its strangely plastic imagery, when given material form, has the power of exciting sensation as well as intuition."[18]

When it speaks to a man in all his parts and functions the symbol has a stirring and life-giving meaning. This is no longer the case when the symbol has ceased to be a living thing. Then it is no longer capable, for instance, of embracing consciousness and the unconscious in one, and it may happen that though the conscious mind "believes" in the value of a certain symbol, the unconscious is pursuing quite a different course. Thus, one can "believe" in the divinity of Christ because this is held to be the supreme revelation of divine love, and at the same time burn everybody as a heretic who does not share that belief—at which Christ himself would have wondered not a little. Heresy-hunts and inquisitions in any form are invariably a sign of one's own unconscious doubt. Torquemada had all the heretics he could lay hands on inquisited and condemned, but the one aim he never reached was the conquest of the—unconscious—doubt in his own soul. A faith like this may regard the *sacrificium intellectus* as a service rendered to God, but it no longer has any experience of the living symbol in the objects it invokes and worships—or purports to worship; for such a faith fights for the maintenance of symbols that are dead to it.

The symbol must also be distinguished from the symptom, for there are certain products of the unconscious which are very similar to symbols. A man does one

[18] *Ibid.*, p. 680.

thing and in reality means another. For instance, the neurotic or psychotic will undertake a lengthy and seemingly unintelligible ceremonial before going to bed. Analysis has shown that these performances have a latent meaning. But they spring from purely unconscious motives that are not at all clear to the performer and are recognized as meaningful only after long and wearisome analytical treatment which may arouse his resistance. The actions are often of a compulsive character, but the person concerned does them without the slightest understanding of what they mean. Yet the moment the unconscious meaning is made conscious, the action loses its compulsive character and ceases to be practised. The conscious mind, therefore, has no part in actions of this kind, not even in the shape of that "feeling" or presentiment which is often bound up with the effect of the symbol; and once the meaning of the symptom has been recognized, it disappears. Such symptoms sometimes resemble the symbolic acts of religion, but their psychological meaning is very different.

"Owing to its nature, the symbol can come to birth only in an alert, highly developed mind, never in one that is dull or lazy. The latter will content itself with the extant symbols given by tradition. Only the passionate yearnings of a keen and cultured mind can create new symbols, the mind not satisfied that the traditional symbols express the highest union. Because the symbol is born of a man's last and highest spiritual attainments and must at the same time include all that is deepest in his nature, it cannot spring exclusively from the most highly differentiated spiritual functions but will in the same measure take its rise from the lowest and most primitive motions of his psyche. For this collaboration of extreme contraries to be possible at all, they must both stand side by side in full and conscious opposition. Such a state will inevitably produce a most violent dichotomy of the self, to the point where thesis and antithesis constantly negate one another, while all the time the ego has unreservedly to recognize the share it has in both. . . . Should a complete equality of opposites be reached . . . the will must come to a standstill; nothing more can be willed, because every motive entails its counter-motive. But as life can never tolerate a standstill, there will be a stoppage of life-energy, and this would lead to an unendurable state of affairs did not the tension of opposites give rise to a new and unitive function leading beyond the opposites. This function comes naturally enough from the regression of libido occasioned by the stoppage. The dichotomy of will has made further progress impossible, so the libido streams off backwards, the river returns to its source: with the immobilization and inactivity of consciousness activity passes to the unconscious, where all differentiated functions have their common archaic root and where we find that mingling of contents of which the primitive mentality still shows numerous traces. The activity of the unconscious now throws up a content which is constellated by thesis and antithesis equally and acts compensatorily to both. Since this content is related to both alike, it forms a kind of middle ground where the opposites can unite." [19] The unconscious expression "forms a raw material which has not to be reduced, but rather shaped and processed and made the common term for thesis and antithesis. In this way it becomes a new content, which now dominates the whole attitude, heals the split, and forces the energy of the opposites into a common river-bed. The stoppage of life is released; life can flow on with strength renewed and to new goals." [20]

[19] *Ibid.*, p. 681.   87   [20] *Ibid.*, p. 681.

The new "expression" coming from the unconscious proves superior to the life-aims so far cherished. It strengthens and sharpens the individuality of all who experience this psychological process. The fresh raw material to be processed by thesis and antithesis Jung calls "the unifying symbol," and the whole of the psychic process that gives rise to it he calls "the transcendental function." Allusions to this symbol-creating process are to be found in the scanty accounts of the initiation-periods undergone by the founders of religion, for instance, in the conflict of Jesus and Satan, Buddha and Mara, Luther and the devil, Zwingli and his worldly past, Faust and Mephistopheles. The symbol-creating process can of course fail, especially when the antithesis is not fully acknowledged. There is an example of this in Nietzsche's *Zarathustra*, where the "Ugliest Man" is suppressed.

The symbol now serves as a goad and the mainspring of conflict for a long time. Almost anything can be used as material for the symbol, in accordance with the fundamental psychological law that anything can be expressed by anything. A gesture, a natural object can be as good a symbol as a product of art. The majority of effective and generally recognized symbols have all assimilated something of the archetypes.

In our account of the transcendental function, we have described what Jung calls "the primordial religious experience." It is not for nothing that he mentions the founders of religion as examples of this. In these cases, too, the predominant rôle falls to the unconscious, for it is from the unconscious that the unifying symbol rises up as an experience to which our human will and instinct can contribute nothing. We can even venture to say that the decisive factor is "pathos" in its original sense of "suffering," i.e. letting things happen: for it can

88

never be seen in advance just what the content of the new symbol will be.

The significance Jung attaches to the unconscious in religious experience will probably not be accepted by everybody without qualification. All theologies, including the Protestant, are sceptical about the unconscious. We have seen that mediaeval Catholicism still recognized dreams as possible sources of revelation, and how this view is no longer accepted in practice. In many of its branches Protestantism is inclined to divorce revelation from psychic experience, or at least not to associate it with psychic life as ordinarily understood. Where it has any knowledge of the unconscious at all, it holds fast to Jung's saying that the unconscious contains all sorts of things that the decent person would rather not face. It is hard indeed to acknowledge that this is the very place from which revelation and the primordial religious experience may come to us, for, as the long procession of psychopaths in the history of church and sect amply proves, it is from the unconscious also that all manner of pseudo-religious garbage has been unloaded on the world. It is easy to understand that a man like Antoni Unternährer [21] was guided by the promptings of his unconscious, which is all the more reason for wishing to hold aloof from it and clinging to the view that the highest religious experiences should not be connected with the unconscious in any way.

From the standpoint of Jungian psychology, we can understand this train of thought, but not accept it. For the term "unconscious" implies no judgement of value. The unconscious is, as we know, the place that contains everything that can possibly be imagined. Things that are differentiated in the conscious mind and can be kept

[21] [A religious fanatic.—Trans.]

89

apart are side by side in the unconscious region of the soul. Unconscious means "not-conscious," but no inferiority in respect of consciousness is thereby expressed. Jung would contend that though the unconscious is an ambiguous and dangerous thing, the same can be said of religious experience. The New Testament says: "It is a fearful thing to fall into the hands of the living God." An apocryphal saying of our Lord runs: "He who is near to me is near to the fire." The religious sage who was asked how one could rise up to God replied: "Those rise up to God who bend low." Above and below go together in religious experience to a larger extent than seems possible to the intellect—and the same is true of the soul.

In this connexion another question will probably be asked which we must also take up here: what is the significance of *spirit* in Jung's psychology? The question is not easy to answer, because Jung very seldom speaks of spirit in his literary work. In one instance he expresses himself as follows: "From the psychological point of view the phenomenon of spirit, like every autonomous complex, appears as an *intention* of the unconscious which is superior to, or at least on a par with, the ego-consciousness. If we are to be fair to what we call spirit we must speak of a higher consciousness rather than of the unconscious; for the very notion of spirit always has the effect of making us associate it with the idea of something superior to ego-consciousness. This superiority is not imputed to spirit as the result of any conscious cogitation, but attaches to it like some essential quality, as is evident from the testimonies of all ages, beginning with the Scripture and ending with Nietzsche's *Zarathustra*. Spirit manifests itself psychologically as a personal being, at times attaining to almost visionary clarity. In Christian dogma it is no less than the third Person of the Trinity. These facts show that spirit is not always merely an idea that can be put into words, but, in its strongest and most immediate revelations, something that exhibits a peculiar life of its own which is felt like that of some being wholly independent of us. So long as spirit is designated and circumscribed by some rational principle or expressible idea, it is not felt as an independent being. But when the idea or principle of it passes beyond our range of vision, when its intentions are lost in the darkness of origin and end, and yet strain towards accomplishment, then spirit is perforce felt as an independent being, as a sort of higher consciousness, and its incalculable and sublime nature can no longer be expressed in terms of human understanding. Our expressive faculties then avail themselves of other means: they devise a symbol." [22] The spirit that reaches out for a symbol in order to express itself is a psychic complex full of creative beginnings and immense possibilities. As an example of the creative spirit Jung cites the spirit of Christianity prevailing in the second century, calling it one of unequalled creativeness. That is why this spirit was felt to be something superior and divine. The moment the spirit begins to promote life it can be described as a sort of higher consciousness transcending our everyday ideals. It is obvious that spirit in this sense ought never to be confused with intellect. Jung also speaks of a spirit that is destructive of life, and this has no right to the title of divinity. The essential criterion is the relation of spirit to life. There is an infatuation which would like to sacrifice all life to spirit because of its superior creativity, and spirit of this kind is a malignant growth that senselessly destroys the living. "Life is the criterion of the

[22] *SPG*, pp. 396 *et seq.*

spirit's truth. A spirit that carries a man beyond the bare possibility of life and seeks fulfilment only in itself is a false spirit—not that the man in question is blameless, since he had it in his power either to give himself up to it or not. Life and spirit are two forces or necessities, and man is placed between them. Spirit endows his life with meaning and the possibility of large developments. But life is indispensable to spirit, for the truth of the spirit is nothing if it cannot live." [23]

Accordingly, Jung allows the spirit two functions: the power to create and the power to experience meaning. Spirit comes from the creative depths of the soul, from those regions which the ego does not touch. In them man experiences a meaning that transcends him. If therefore spirit comes from beyond consciousness, i.e. from the unconscious, we are tempted to put it like this: spirit comes from the supra-conscious, the psychic realm that is above the conscious mind. Jung, however, defines the unconscious simply as that which is not conscious. He purposely never uses the term "sub-conscious." He attaches not the slightest *valuation* to the idea of the unconscious and leaves the question completely open whether the unconscious is above or below consciousness. He is to be taken as saying that the unconscious is as much below it as above. Hence, in Jung's sense, spirit is endued simply with the quality of the unconscious. At the same time a distinction must be made between it and the other contents of the unconscious—nature, for instance. Although it is nowhere explicitly stated in the passages we have quoted from Jung, it is implied that spirit liberates us from the "natural" impulses of life and can lead us to shape life on a higher plane. In this freedom there is also the possibility of spirit turning against

[23] *Ibid.*, p. 400.

life, thus becoming the antagonist of life and the soul. But this antagonistic attitude is a bare possibility, not a necessity. Jung rejects the interpretation of spirit to be found in Ludwig Klages's philosophy and teachings concerning the soul, in so far as these ascribe to spirit an unqualified enmity to life.

On an earlier page we used the image of the individual's consciousness as an island emerging from the ocean of the unconscious, with man thus bedded in a psychic reality that far transcends him as an individual. We must now modify this image and say, perhaps, that the upward movement of the emerging island is caused by supra-personal and unconscious forces—the spiritual forces which carry a man beyond his "natural" element and put him in touch with processes occurring in the world of meaning and the world of the spirit. This is about as far as pictures will go in giving Jung's idea. All pictures are to be employed only with the greatest circumspection in psychology, and always in the realization that their figurative way of expressing what one means is an improper way. Pictures and images adhere to a dimensional framework, and in the world of the psyche there are no dimensions: above and below do not exist in the ordinary sense. Nor do they exist in religion either. Religious symbolism often sets the sublimest things and the most crudely sensual side by side, sometimes even expressing the one by means of the other. In this respect Indian temples offer examples that are as instructive as they are surprising, and the same is true of the Christian Gnostics and, occasionally, Christian art and symbolism. Those who are still not satisfied should read what Jesus has to say in the Gospels about the above and the below. They will soon see that Jesus regarded our fine distinctions in these matters as merely human ways of looking at things, but that before God it was very different. All religion, Christianity included, is in this sense as revolutionary and irrational as we could possibly desire.

Speaking figuratively again, Jung sees man harnessed between that which has not yet attained to consciousness and that which is above consciousness. The "natural" ground of our being as well as the spirit both affect consciousness, but in different ways; and only through the experience of both realms together are we made men. He calls both of them unconscious. We must therefore be quite clear in our minds that this unconscious is, in Jung's sense, a highly antithetical quantity uniting in itself all manner of contents and functions, and that the term "unconscious" is far from expressing a valuation, only a relationship in respect of consciousness. Religious experience, in particular, contains elements of the naturalistic psyche as well as of the spirit; hence it unites man with his archaic origins and the naturalistic basis of his being, and yet by its spiritual function enables him to transcend himself. In the last resort the unconscious carries out the truth of the old saying: *natura naturam vincit*.

It is therefore absolutely understandable why religious experience is, for Jung, so closely connected with the unconscious. All sorts of objections may be raised against this view, yet when we examine the few allusions in the New Testament to the pentecostal experience, in the light of Jung's insight, much is made clearer and intelligible. The notion that in many religious phenomena we are dealing with supra-personal forces which wield a fate-like power over our lives is indeed very probable. Since they lie on the further side of the ego, they are forces of the unconscious, using the word in the Jungian sense, with no idea of "sub-conscious" at the back of it. It is rather conceived as the aggregate of all psychic events occurring *beyond consciousness*, where the lowest is one with the highest, and where we reach the end of all knowledge and nothing remains for us but to marvel at the sublime.

RELIGION AS A PSYCHIC FUNCTION

ODERN psychology, particularly analytical psychology, is not content simply to point out the various psychic elements contained in religion. It is also concerned with the question of what the function of religion is in the individual's personality, what place it has in man's psyche as a whole.

Fundamentally, this question is not so far removed from theology, for in practice it too must concern itself with the problem: what does religion mean, and what should it offer, to people in general? The theologian who indulges in apologetics and defends his faith against hostile attacks is faced with the somewhat tricky problem of making religion plausible to his fellows. Protestant theology has been working away at this theme ever since the end of orthodoxy. The Age of Enlightenment stressed the utility of religion; pietism held out happiness. Both introduced a eudaemonistic principle into the Christian message. Today we have given up this view because of its triteness. But in some way or other we want to make religion and particularly Christianity acceptable, and the most frequently used arguments all aim at showing that religion satisfies a need. In theology itself the "need-theory" has taken the form of the so-called theory of value: whatever satisfies a need is valuable, and value is the guarantee of truth. If therefore a religion can satisfy the religious need, its value is thereby proved and at the same time its inner truth.

Appearing in the guise of sermons and edifying literature, this need-theory appeals to man's sense of imperfection, or, more recently, to his fear of life. "You have here a way of satisfying your feeling of imperfection; you will be rid of your fear of life if you believe. Well then, believe—i.e. accept the doctrine we proclaim." This appeal is applied with more or less skill and tact, according to the verve of the individual preacher and the educational level of the community he represents.

People are anxious to know what modern psychology has to say on the subject. On this point—Christianity's message—theology comes closest in its work to psychology. We postulate a religious need. If there really is such a thing, then psychology will assuredly know something about it. People are therefore anxious to know whether psychology will confirm this argument of theology or whether things are different.

Approaching this question from the point of view of Jung's psychology, we must say at once that the real situation is in fact different. There are, of course, psychic facts which can be interpreted as religious need. There is also a connection between fear of life and religion, but when the two are coupled together as in official Church propaganda (and in that of many sects), all that this short-circuiting procedure reveals is a complete lack of insight into the human soul as it really is.

What, then, is the psychic function of religion?

If we are to answer this question in the Jungian sense as broadly as possible, we must first go back to what we have said already, namely, that religion is inner experience; that it contains a great many experiences of our unconscious psyche; and that in them we are often dealing with supra-personal psychic contents and forces. We have also stated that all psychic experience is really "pathos"—suffering, letting things happen. The supra-personal forces of the soul—the unconscious with all its enigmas and ambiguities—come over us like fate. They come over us without our being able to say anything about it, without the possibility of our inducing or avoiding it. We must now modify this view. Psychic processes can be experienced in two ways—actively or passively. When a man experiences certain contents of his psyche passively only, they pass over him and influence him, but he is merely pushed about by them. A man who experiences them actively, however, is able to give them a certain direction; he is not just pushed about in the psychic process, he actively intervenes in it and can, for instance, give it a meaning. We all know from practical experience, psychology apart, that it is not the same thing for a man to bury his guilt and remorse in himself or to get it out in a confession. A man who knows that he has incurred guilt and that it is "biting" him, but who stops at that, will develop his personality very differently from one who "gets it off his chest" by confessing. By confessing we are not thinking solely of the Catholic confessional; confession can easily consist in reparation of the wrong before the person wronged, or in any other form of open acknowledgement of the guilt. At all events, the individual does not remain passive if he experiences guilt and remorse in this way. He wins to greater self-knowledge than the man who simply lets the experience cripple him. This possibility of taking an active part in psychic events is given to us from the start. We can put it figuratively like this: the individual can let himself drift in the river of psychic occurrence, he can even let himself sink in it and take the consequences—or he can maintain a certain direction in mid stream, like a swimmer. As in genuine rivers, it is difficult to swim against the psychic current, but within certain bounds a man's activity can intervene decisively. (N.B.: Though this comparison is simply an image, and ought not to be pressed or interpreted too far, it gives us a tolerably clear idea of the state of affairs we mean.)

This is where religion comes in, for in the last analysis religion consists not in merely experiencing the suprapersonal forces of the soul as such, but in adopting—psychically—an active attitude. This can happen in various ways, with very different attitudes and distinct ends in view; and the final result will differ accordingly. But the basic principle is that the complete personality should engage in a living, psychically active encounter with the forces dwelling in the soul, or rather with the forces we meet in our inward experience.

Trying now to explain in detail what we mean, we shall find it best to begin with the religious act itself—the rite. It is fairly obvious that man wants to exert some kind of influence here. On the face of it the object of this influence is a part of his surroundings. Among primitive peoples the idea of *mana* bulks large: mysterious, omnipresent energy. According to Jung, *mana* is a projection of libido or psychic energy, and the meaning of the ritual act consists in trying to canalize the libido in a certain direction. Thus Jung interprets the sacrifice of a horse as a measure designed to suppress backwards-looking libido in favour of forward-looking libido.[1] Animal sacrifice means the sacrificing of the animalistic, i.e. sexual, libido,[2] thus facilitating a turning towards cultural work. All ritual tries to displace libido when it is no longer desirable that interest should be fastened on a certain object.[3] Thus, the initiation of youths tries to

[1] *WSL*, p. 448.   [2] *Ibid.*, p. 45.   [3] *UES*, p. 72.

draw libido away from the mother.[4] Everything connected with this initiation clearly aims at the separation from the mother, and, positively, at the adoption of a new attitude. The "mysteries," too, aim at releasing a certain psychic event in man, and they certainly succeed as long as the religion in question is a living one. The "incest-wish" plays a big part here, that is to say, the wish to return to the mother. This is not, however, simply a matter of what we would regard as abnormal or perverted sexuality in the sense intended by Freud. The incest-wish undoubtedly existed at one time, as the strict taboos show that had to be raised up against it during certain phases of man's development. But the reason for this wish to get back to the womb is that the womb is the symbol of psychic collectivity. At the back of it is man's knowledge of the pain involved in developing a consciousness and an ego. It was far from easy for prehistoric man to become a separate personality—as neurotics prove, it is not very easy today either. The incest-wish appears as a reaction that had to be overcome by taboos. Jung supposes that the Eleusinian Mysteries were designed to overcome this wish.[5] The psychic mechanism is as follows: A fantasy is activated which brings about the detachment of the mother-image from the real mother. In this way the mother is spiritualized together with the libido attaching to her. The spiritualized libido can then be carried over into cultural activities.[6]

In Christianity too we come across similar spiritualizations of libido. By way of example Jung tells us how the cult of courtly love in the Middle Ages changed into the cult of the soul, setting a portion of libido free for cultural work. This example indicates that there are

[4] BZIU, p. 133.   [5] WSL, p. 372.   [6] Ibid., p. 268.

limits to man's canalization of libido. It is, psychologically speaking, no accident that with the rise of this cult of the soul witch-hunting also appears—that dread scourge of the Middle Ages and the Renaissance. It arose because part of the libido sinks back into the unconscious and activates unconscious complexes which then emerge into consciousness and begin to function there.[7]

Religious ceremonies are ultimately only a psychic preparation for work.[8] As an example Jung refers to fertility magic. Primitive religion knows this in the most obvious and purely sexual form: copulation in the field. In the spring the peasant and his wife come together in their field so as to increase its fertility. Later the natural act is replaced by a symbolical one, the sprinkling with holy water: the libido is carried over from crude naturalism into cultural activity. In this connexion Jung makes the interesting aside that the "sexual question" only arises in towns and factories, not among the peasantry, because agricultural work partly desexualizes libido and, through its natural symbolism, transforms the latter into strength for work, which is not the case with mechanical and factory labour. At any rate, ritual always serves to set free the libido which man needs for his work.[9]

It is really implicit in what we have said already that an intimate tie exists between religion and man's psychic state, for the canalization of libido must follow very different rules with primitive and with civilized man. But this is true also in another sense. As we have seen earlier, the religious functions are closely connected with the unconscious; and in Jung's view the unconscious is compensatory to consciousness. It brings the "Absolutely

[7] *PT*, p. 331.   [8] *WSL*, p. 440.   [9] *PT*, p. 297 n.

Other" to bear—that of which consciousness in its momentary states takes no account. Consequently, religion too has a compensatory significance in respect of man's consciousness and his psychological state. Hence religion does not remain the same everywhere but varies as to its content with the psychic state of a people as a whole. This is as true of the different religions as of a single religion in the different phases of its development. We can go so far as to say that religion has a different meaning for the individual according to his age. Such ideas can be verified by theological research, since even the briefest glimpse into primitive Christianity will reveal the enormous difference between the religious experience of an early Christian and that of a Protestant today. There are also marked differences between religious feeling now and in the age of the Reformation; and one would have to go very deep to find in the two thousand years of Christianity a basic principle that was everywhere present and the same.

Jung adduces proofs for his thesis from every field of religious history. In the case of primitive religion its starting-point is the characteristic fact that primitive man is a wholly collective being. He has scarcely awakened to his "I-ness"—hence this is still very much imperilled.[10] The contents of the collective unconscious and of the collective psyche are always on the verge of invading the soul and destroying the ego. That is why primitive man is constantly in danger of running amuck or succumbing to psychic catastrophes of that kind. But since religion is compensatory to the conscious situation, its aim is to help him consolidate his ego.[11] Religion safeguards primitive man against the perils of the soul. Primitive cosmogony as recounted in myths is really a

[10] *BZlU*, p. 50; *PT*, p. 20; *SPG*, p. 168.   [11] *EJ 1934*, p. 201.

psychic cosmogony, i.e. the image of how consciousness arose and is consolidated.[12] Primitive man's soul contains many foreign bodies that he is incapable of assimilating. Here too religion affords the necessary help by objectifying these psychic contents as demons, spirits of the dead, etc. and thus enabling them to be divorced from the ego and extruded from the soul. In this way they cease to be dangerous in so far as after their objectification the ego can no longer be disintegrated or possessed by them.[13] The objectification and projection of contents which the ego cannot assimilate without grave danger to itself is an absolute necessity for the primitive soul and an act of psychic hygiene,[14] otherwise primitive man could not withstand the danger and would soon lose his ego.

The primitive soul is also characterized by a marked *attachment to the object.* He sees himself in others and in the things of the surrounding world, and can thus only partially distinguish himself from it and the various objects in it.[15] This condition of *participation mystique,* as Jung calls it following Lévy-Brühl, is marked by the expectation that whatever happens outside me will also happen inside me, and conversely that I shall be able to find the processes going on inside me, in the surrounding world.[16] In this state of imperfect differentiation between subject and object the objective psyche must be repressed.[17] This is an absolute necessity and is achieved through the objectification of the non-assimilable contents of the soul, e.g. dreams. Such contents, objectified, give rise to the belief in spirits, as also do visions, diseases

[12] *WSL*, p. 445.   [13] *UES*, pp. 175, 201.
[14] *Das Unbewusste im normalen und kranken Seelenleben*, p. 103.
[15] *UES*, p. 169.   [16] *SPG*, p. 168.   [17] *BZIU*, p. 50.

of the mind, etc.[18] In this way it is possible for primitive man to free himself from the objective psyche and protect his own ego. Religious magic enables him to influence these alien contents. Jung calls it the "night-religion of primitives," [19] by which he probably means that man can thereby control and exorcize certain elements in his soul. All the complexes and alien psychic contents are thus exposed to man's observation and understanding, and he himself is rid of the danger of possession they harbour for his ego. His ego-consciousness becomes clearer and firmer, so that primitive religion is a stage on the way to self-consciousness. The psychological mechanism is the same as with civilized man. Just as the latter rids himself of certain psychic contents with the aid of confession, and on the other hand uses philosophy and religion in order to come to terms with his inner world, so primitive man uses magic.[20]

We should not leave primitive religion without expressly remarking that civilized man even in the twentieth century is not without his share in it, firstly in the sense that in our development from childhood onwards, we all go through phases which clearly reveal certain primitive characteristics,[21] but also in the sense that every adult person still bears the traces of an earlier frame of mind in his very nature. Jung quotes Nietzsche's idea that in dreams we go through the earlier stages of human development. Thus, the primitive mentality is not altogether overcome in us, only built over by a new one. Proof of this is the fact that we can still find features in present-day civilization that clearly hark back to the primitive view of the world. Illusion can therefore still exercise its power, which, according to Jung, is the magic

<hr>

[18] *PT*, p. 45; *UES*, p. 200.
[19] *SPG*, p. 182.
[20] *Ibid.*, p. 174.
[21] *WSL*, p. 230.

power of the word.[22] The idea of man as a microcosm which corresponds to the macrocosm rests on the last traces of an original psychic identity.[23] Neither is psychic objectivity a new idea, since ultimately it tallies with the primitive belief in ghosts.[24] The idealization of certain things, too, is analogous to the primitive objectification of psychic facts: we idealize that which we want to exorcize—a procedure called "apotropaism."[25] In view of all this, Jung thinks that he is justified in concluding that modern man is fundamentally archaic.[26] Primitive man is just as logical as we are, only he starts from different assumptions.[27] He ascribes everything that happens to an arbitrary power,[28] which at bottom we also believe in. He projects his undifferentiated soul into his environment, whence arises his belief in spirits.[29] In the last analysis, our religious thinking is still primitive thinking.[30] Indeed, Jung holds that particularly as regards religion the primitive mentality is still very much in evidence with us. Here Jung voices an idea to which we shall return later on, namely that Western man is still a barbarian where his soul is concerned, a fact that redounds to his ill.

However, Jung does not, in the manner of the all-simplifying "scientist," reduce the great religions of civilization to primitive ritual. Although he may stress that vestiges of the archaic attitude are to be found in our religious life, he still sees that the task of the civilized religion, and particularly Christianity, is modified by the psychic situation of civilized man. The civilized religion no longer has to reckon with a weak ego-function. Civilized man's consciousness is sufficiently strong not to be overwhelmed so easily by unconscious contents and

[22] PT, p. 64.
[23] EI 1937, p. 40.
[24] BZIU, p. 112.
[25] EI 1938, p. 441.
[26] SPG, p. 212.
[27] Ibid., p. 212.
[28] Ibid., p. 220.
[29] Ibid., p. 237.
[30] Ibid., p. 240.

thus put out of action. On the other hand, it is subject to other compulsions.

Jung sees the law of psychological compensation operating in Christianity as well. For him, the religion of the West is Christianity, and he has accordingly devoted the greatest attention to it. Neither a Germanic religion, nor the Graeco-Roman religion of the last days of antiquity, nor any other religion could be, in Jung's eyes, the religion of the West, but Christianity and Christianity alone. Judging by his knowledge of Western man, he sees no reason to assume that any other religion would be more suited to the West than Christianity. This positive attitude to Christianity does not, however, prevent him from expressing himself with complete lack of prejudice in his judgements or from carrying out his researches impartially; and not everybody who confesses Christianity in one form or another will feel happy or satisfied with what Jung has to say on individual questions.

Obviously, Christianity is not a fixed quantity for Jung, something that has fallen ready-made from Heaven and has no links with its environment: the last days of antiquity. As we have already intimated, the law of psychological compensation holds good for Christianity too. It is, first of all, a compensation for the slavery that was fundamental to the economic life of the time.[31] Secondly, it is the negative side of the classical cult of sex. The last days of antiquity knew an unparalleled sexual licence. Consequently, there arose by way of compensation a religion that repressed sex and regarded it as inferior; inevitably therefore it championed asceticism. It may be that many will question this interpretation. For the "sexual question" as it had been known in Palestine

[31] *Die Frau in Europa*, p. 23.

did not exist in primitive Christianity, because people were expecting the end of the world at any moment. But if Jung's interpretation is not true of Jesus and, possibly, Paul, it certainly is true of Augustine; for it was not the eschatological expectations of the early days that were now shaping Christianity but the sort of thinking and feeling that had the closest ties with all the lights and shadows of the Greco-Roman world, and this was crystallized in St. Augustine. Also, for many people other than Christians various phenomena at that time were becoming problems and occasioning attempts at reform. Thus the Stoics were tackling the problem of slavery. All these separate elements drew together in the nascent Catholic Church, so that as sole representative of the Christianity of the age she became at once the heir to, and conqueror of, her times.

This is also true of specifically religious factors. Like Mithraism, Christianity agreed that a sacrifice was demanded of man. This demand followed from the psychic situation inherent in the twilight of antiquity, which both sought and required a taming of the instincts.[32] But Mithraism demanded only the sacrifice of the instincts themselves, whereas Christianity demanded the sacrifice of the whole man,[33] which accounts for the superiority of the latter. It devalued sexuality; in its worship and ritual it transferred the libido to other objects, thereby discovering the value of personality.[34] It is therefore no accident that we can date the beginnings of modern psychology from St. Augustine's *Confessions*—the same Augustine who, as bishop, indulged in such impressive encomiums on the subject of virginity. At any rate, the acquisition of Christian values demanded a high price of man. For Jung, Mithraism is only a stopgap, since it always led the libido back to nature and was

32 *WSL*, p. 185.   33 *Ibid.*, p. 458.   34 *Ibid.*, pp. 270, 274.

therefore extraverted.[35] Christianity went further and released man from his natural bonds, disengaged him from his instincts. Only in this way could that higher consciousness be attained which is the boon of Christianity.[36] It achieved this through a marked other-worldliness and regard for the future. The old thinking was, on the contrary, essentially retrospective.[37] Hence a completely new attitude arose which necessarily brought with it a new level of consciousness. This in its turn effected one of the great transformations of the collective psyche.

Another of the compensatory workings of religion is that it prepares man for death. Death is the obverse of life. Buddhism as well as Christianity teaches this preparation for dying. Death is no problem for man so long as he is psychically contained in the collectivity. There are then no dead in the sense that life has ceased for them, but the dead continue to exist as spirits, and may even come back to life in a rebirth. Many primitive peoples take it for granted that a man is reborn in his grandchild. But when a man's personality and ego are more fully developed, death will appear in quite another way, always provided that he remains conscious of his ego. Then death is definitely the end of a certain state; hence religion on this spiritual level must regard death quite otherwise than does primitive religion.[38] That is why Christianity was able to reorient the classical outlook and turn its attention to the Beyond.

Religions also convey an experience of the transcendental side of life, as, for instance, in the Catholic Mass;[39] but the mystery-cults too prepare man for an afterlife.[40] By this, however, they understand not only a Beyond in the Catholic sense of another world, but a Beyond of

[35] Ibid., p. 189.
[36] SPG, p. 250.
[37] PT, p. 120.
[38] WS, p. 219.
[39] EJ 1939, p. 406.
[40] Bardo Thödol, p. 21.

deliverance and a Beyond of consciousness. Jung takes *transcendence* to mean something different from what is meant in philosophy; it is something beyond consciousness, beyond our present psychic constellation. At any rate, religion offers man the knowledge of new spiritual possibilities which may be realized, for instance, through a "rebirth"; it discloses the "Absolutely Other" that transcends all previous attitudes and the existing state of personality. Closely connected with this is the fact that the mysteries always "link back" to the original sources of life and strength.[41] In this respect the task of religion is to do what the symbol does: bring opposites together. It ought to contain life's Absolutely Other. The highest and the lowest go together. But if a church fails to bring them together, a sect will instantly spring up, or some kind of underground movement, which thereupon takes charge of this. The Catholic Church has, in the popular mind, some such connexion with subterranean forces in the figure of the shrewd Capuchin. Protestantism fares rather worse in this respect, but it was not by mere chance that the legendary figure of Dr. Faustus appeared together with Martin Luther. It would seem that compensation is the function of religion and that in the end it always strives to bring about man's wholeness. Religion embraces the whole of a man, and the whole man will always come to the fore in the religious situation of his age, whether this wholeness expresses itself in a single religious community of the most comprehensive character imaginable, as in mediaeval Catholicism, or in a multiplicity of religious movements and communities all engaged in realizing some rightful theme.

Adolf Keller, in his exposition of Jung's religious psy-

[41] *EJ 1935*, p. 40.

chology mentioned at the beginning of this book, places Jung side by side with the dialectical theologian Karl Barth, because Jung stresses the fact that religion serves to make man conscious of the Absolutely Other. As is well known, Barth interprets Christianity as resting on supernatural revelation, which revelation, he says, is the Absolutely Other, that which is unproportioned to reality in every respect. When Keller wrote his treatise it was probably more justifiable than it is today to mention Jung in the same breath as Barth. But even then it must have been obvious that the two men meant totally different things by the same word. For Barth the Absolutely Other has nothing whatever to do with the reality in which we live, and it is only given us to know it in supernatural revelation. According to Barth's theology, the Absolutely Other is neither accessible to man save on the assumption of revelation, nor is it in the last resort experienceable. How it is possible for a man to have knowledge of an Absolutely Other and talk and write about it without being able to experience it is not very clear; it is a statement for which Barth himself must accept responsibility. But it is patent to everybody who is at all familiar with Barth's thought that he strongly opposes any form of experiential or empirical theology, and for this reason it is incomprehensible how Keller, who certainly knows Barth the theologian, comes to equate him with Jung. For according to Jung, the thing that he once happened to designate by the term Absolutely Other is definitely experienceable. It is a psychologically definable quantity, and his aim is to demonstrate the effect it has in transforming the personality. The individual is transformed by it in an empirically demonstrable way. This is something that Barth from his point of view would never concede for his theological concept of the Absolutely Other; and if, in his eyes, theology and philosophy cannot have anything to say about it, because it is beyond their grasp, the same will also be true of psychology.

Now that we have cleared this matter up, let us return to Jung. In his view the experience of the Absolutely Other, once religion has brought it near and enabled a man to have it, is expressed in the process of rebirth or redemption. The struggle for rebirth is age old, for in it is voiced man's wish for a renewal of life. It is not only Christianity that speaks of dying and rising again; the theme appears in all religions, and we might well call rebirth an archetype. In his early work *Psychology of the Unconscious*, Jung deals with rebirth and says that it is possible for man to attain it by turning within. In this way the libido "introverts" and brings about a renewal of life.

Jung returns to this theme later, among other places in a lecture delivered at the Eranos Conference in 1939,[42] where he says that rebirth is a purely psychic affair [43] and one of the primordial utterances of man. It has two roots: knowledge of the transcendental element in life and the experience of a change in man's own being.[44] Rebirth, however, is not of uniform aspect. It may have to do with metempsychosis (transmigration of souls) or reincarnation (resurrection) or rebirth within the span of an individual's life (regeneration). It can occur with or without a change in his nature (transmutation). The change can come from his taking part in some ritual process of transformation.[45] Subjective changes can take the form of a diminution of

---

[42] *EJ 1939.*
[43] *Ibid.,* p. 404.
[44] *Ibid.,* p. 406.
[45] *Ibid.,* p. 404.

personality or loss of soul or increase of personality. As an example of the last, Jung cites Paul. An event of this kind can take place in connexion with the Christ-symbol, in which mortality and immortality are one.[46] There may also be an inner structural change, for instance in possession, where a man is consumed in his persona or identifies himself with an ancestor. Similarly, he can identify himself with a group or with a "culture-hero." Magical processes too can induce a change of personality, likewise technical procedures such as yoga or the *exercitia spiritualia* of Ignatius Loyola. Finally, the possibility of inner change can come from natural processes, which make themselves felt as influences emanating from the unconscious: the "Other," or the Other *in us*, asserts itself, and its voice may in certain circumstances be regarded as the voice of God. We shall deal with these processes when we come to the process of individuation.

Jung has also gone into the question of the great changes in consciousness that may be brought about by the renunciation of selfhood in mysticism.[47] It leads ultimately to a new work of selfhood, as the hints of the mystics show. What is demanded is an inner freedom from all images, so that the individual can turn inwards and hear God's voice (Ruysbroek). In that state the effects of objects no longer impinge on an ego-bound consciousness, but an altogether different effect is reached which has the ego not for a subject but for an object. Jung quotes Paul's saying: "Yet not I, but Christ liveth in me: and the life which I now live in the flesh, I live by the faith of the Son of God, who loved me, and gave

[46] *Ibid.,* p. 410.
[47] Jung-Suzuki: *Die grosse Befreiung,* p. 19.

himself for me" (Gal. ii. 20). Thus a new state of consciousness is produced which cannot be apprehended by thought in its final reaches, but can only be striven after on the ground of religion.

Of all these themes it is *individuation* that has absorbed Jung most, the natural road to rebirth; and our task now is to show what this individuation can mean to people.

Jung's latest publications all relate in one way or another to the process of individuation. He finds examples of it in all religions, including the non-Christian ones. The Catholic Mass has to do with individuation, but Jung also finds it as the psychic background to early Christian gnosticism and its heir, alchemy. Individuation is also present in the experiences communicated by the secret societies of China, and it is likewise the aim of the discipline taught by the Zen Buddhist schools of Japan. The name differs, of course, but the spiritual effects and powers which the various processes convey all agree with what our scientific terminology most fittingly describes as individuation. Further, Jung thinks that individuation discloses the process of primordial religious experience, as he calls it; and that what we describe as "the transcendental function"—the aim of which is the crystallization of a new symbol—is, formally speaking, the same process of individuation that we are now trying to grasp in its significance for personality. In it there is a point at which the interests of the psychologist and psychotherapist coincide with those of the student of religion. The more Jung became engrossed in the explanation of this psychic function, the further he penetrated into the field of religious research. It was at this juncture that he met Richard Wilhelm. When Jung, in his investigation of Europeans, first hit on the phenomenon of individuation, it struck him as baffling in the extreme and in its very nature inscrutable, until Wilhelm placed certain material at his disposal dealing with religious life in China, which suddenly threw light on a number of problems.

One must be clear at the outset that the nature of the processes about to be described does not make the task of presenting them any easier. We have to do first and foremost with a highly significant and highly personal experience, which it is far from easy to put into words, let alone describe accurately. Jung says: the best of these experiences cannot be put into words at all, and the second-best misses the mark. Hence the likelihood of misunderstandings is considerable. In order to understand what it is all about, one should have experienced it already, and, for the reasons given below, an experience of this kind is not a matter of course and is therefore rather rare. On the contrary, it is more the normal thing for the great majority of people not to have experienced it. In this respect Jung's psychology is in agreement with what those acquainted with the mystery religions say. At the back of these mysteries too there are very personal and profound psychic processes, the nature of which, however, does not lend itself to everybody's understanding.

Then we must make another observation in order to avoid possible misunderstandings: all the processes and psychological events in question are to be taken *figuratively*. That is to say, they are but the *reflexions* of the events that constitute the essential part of this experience. We know so little about the nature of the psychic events in question that we can say next to nothing about them. All that we have access to are their reflections; they themselves remain inaccessible.

The need for a European to have experience of individuation comes with the problem of the climacteric. Jung is probably the first psychologist to recognize with great clearness that the psychic problems of the young man are not the same as those of the elderly man. The task of the young man he describes as adaptation to the external world in the widest sense. The young man has to make a place for himself in society, in his profession, in marriage and family; he has to acquire and develop all the faculties that will enable him to fill this place. He can do that only by adapting himself as much as possible to the demands of his environment. It is therefore a question, generally speaking, of his struggling to achieve something in life, making a position for himself and winning a "place in the sun." Ultimately, of course, it does not depend on a man's individual decision whether he shall or shall not take up the fight: circumstances drive him to it. He has to win a position of some sort in order to live at all, and this forces him to adapt himself to the world. Also society, the collectivity in which he lives, makes demands on him morally, legally, and spiritually. In general, the need for adaptation develops a special function which Jung calls the *persona* (see above). It is the rôle a man plays in and for the world more or less voluntarily and more or less consciously. The necessity of being active and adapting himself to the demands of the world also compels him to select, from among the faculties at his disposal, the one which seems to offer him most possibilities. That leads, as we have described, to the development of a primary function, then a secondary function among the four functions of thinking, feeling, sensation, and intuition. He takes the one that is most differentiated in him as the primary function and consciously lets it determine and shape him, while the others fall more and more into the unconscious in proportion as they are less developed. The type develops accordingly; and the individual's attitude—whether he is an extravert or an introvert—is the second characteristic by which he may be gauged in respect of his type. All that is not developed falls to the unconscious and hence to that side of a man which now becomes, as it were, his dark double.

The process of adaptation to the world has made him viable, with the result that he can now satisfy its demands. At the same time, however, he has to do not only with an external world but with an internal world as well. And of this he has not taken full account during the process of adaptation. On the contrary: all his energy turned to the external world, and the internal world was patently neglected. Also, the fact that a part of his personality and his psychic faculties fell to the unconscious, the shadow, is a cause of dissatisfaction. By allowing a part of his being to lapse, he fails to become what he really has it in him to become.

Hence, in the second half of life, when the task of the first has been successfully accomplished, another task begins to loom. The individual is compelled to come to terms with his "within," his soul. We can say that what is now demanded is adaptation to the inner world. Outward adaptation is no easy matter, and inward adaptation makes no lesser demands. We are concerned with a very complicated psychic process which engages the whole man and ultimately all his faculties as well.

The pressing need for this process can show itself in any number of ways. A man often feels that his life has suddenly lost all meaning. At the very moment when he has successfully adapted himself to the world and he can say that his life is at its peak, all at once, stealthily, the question comes: what's the use of all this effort? He then discovers that though he is doing all sorts of valuable things, he is unable to say why, and what the point is. His life has lost its meaning. In Jung's experience very successful businessmen of the American type are sometimes faced with a personal crisis of this sort. Another thing that leads up to it is the sudden and unexpected recognition, when one thought that one knew everything, of a side unknown to oneself. The social problem may show us, perhaps, that there is an "above" and a "below." The rich man "discovers" poverty, and not merely as lack of money and possessions but as a hard and hopeless sort of existence that is everlastingly dogged by the relentless struggle for the bare necessities of life. Married couples faced with a similar situation discover sides in one another which were, of course, always there but of which they had no conscious knowledge. In the first years of marriage, so much energy is used up in the creation of economic security that there is no possibility of the couple's becoming a psychological problem to one another, particularly if they are spiritually attuned. But the moment external security has been reached more or less, it suddenly becomes clear that one's partner is quite different from oneself, that one knows nothing about him and cannot understand him. He has become a spiritual problem.

Indeed, a man can easily become a spiritual problem to himself. He discovers that he is not the man he thought he was. Jung relates how a man who had lived in the utmost respectability all his life woke up one night and announced that at bottom he was a morally inferior person and that his virtuousness was nothing but a show, whereupon he spent the remainder of his days in riotous living. This man had hidden his "shadow" from himself and others, and then on discovering it had logically put into practice what appeared to him to be the truth. Even if all men do not go quite so far at this point, experiencing, as it were, a negative conversion, the dark and "morally inferior" side is apt to obtrude itself in the second half of life. All of us are led or rather constrained by society to a certain morality, and for reasons of adaptation we accept it. But once the adaptation has succeeded, one notices that the moral figure one cuts in accordance with the standards of the collectivity does not fit in at all well with one's own personal tendencies, as one had previously thought. A contradiction sets in between what one is and what one is supposed to be.

Ultimately, the problem of the climacteric is the problem of opposites. Our experience of life is that it is somehow based on opposites, and we realize that apart from our present achievements there is something quite different—the Other. The material in or through which a man experiences the opposite is different in each case and is probably related to the attitude or function-type of the individual. But however various the forms may be, it is always a matter of the individual's realizing that the opposite, the Other, exists, and that he is faced with the problem of uniting the opposites.

This problem must now be solved. That it is not easy of solution a single glance into the history of Christian theology will show; for in the battles which theologians waged, and still wage, among themselves the root question more often than not is precisely the union of opposites. We have only to think of the theodicy problem which has exercised the minds of theologians at all times, or the problem of whether God the Redeemer can also be God the Creator. The theodicy problem is concerned with how God is related to evil, whether he is the author of it or whether he only suffers it or how the relationship is to be defined at all. Theologians and non-theologians alike have pondered this question ever since Christianity began, without having found a generally accepted answer so far. One of the latest efforts at solving it in Protestant theology is Karl Barth's idea of the Absolutely Other, which, as originally formulated, did offer the beginnings of an answer. But Barth's subsequent development and that of the theology associated with him have tended in a direction which can scarcely offer any solution whatever, since the whole opposition between God the Creator and the evil of this world is denied in the assertion that God has nothing to do with this life and this reality, because Creation, thanks to the Fall, has passed clean beyond God's reach. With this people think that the world is rid of the theodicy problem—at the cost, however, of God's having nothing to do with either man or reality. That is not, of course, a solution of the problem of opposites, only an evasion of it, which is satisfying neither religiously nor theologically nor philosophically. The old gnosticism tried another solution and hypothecated two gods: a demiurge who created an imperfect world, and a Redeemer who guides the world to perfection. In the wranglings over the doctrine of predestination during and since the Reformation, the same problem arises in the form of the question whether God's will was involved in the Fall of man or not. The reformed churches have ever been notoriously disunited as to the solution of this conflict, and the problems still await solution today. All problems that have to do with opposites are as difficult as they are significant for religion.

When a man becomes conscious of it in his life, it may happen that the problem of opposites appears as a *personal* problem only to a limited extent. In this case, if he is not yet fully conscious of it, he may find the solution in some existing symbol. In speaking of the transcendental function and the resultant constellation of symbols, we saw that these may be of supra-personal significance, i.e. that in the symbol wherein some religious founder experienced the unity transcending the opposites, other people too may find the same. Every traditional religion has such symbols, and many people find what they need in them. When a man discovers the solution to his personal crisis in a traditional symbol such as may be afforded by a rite, a dogma, a form of worship, he experiences this symbol with all the greater intensity, and it becomes inwardly alive for him. Then, though he may change somewhat, his changing, like the crisis itself, is not something of which he is fully conscious. He simply slips through the crisis, or partially slips through, without really discovering what it is all about. The symbol then in fact becomes for him what Jung has so clearly and tellingly described: the expression of something intuited but not made fully conscious. The individual in question also experiences the whole process of change as a redemption.

If, however, he cannot avail himself of a universal symbol, the process must now set in which Jung calls individuation. This road is by no means easy, and Jung is of the opinion that only an inner need justifies a man in taking it. Otherwise the solution afforded by traditional religion is to be preferred. The process is called "individuation" because it brings about the restoration of individuality, of one's own personality. Personality must be enlarged by making conscious an essential part of what has hitherto been unconscious. The aim is not what we commonly mean by "individualism," or even by an "individualistic" way of looking at things, i.e. a markedly egocentric attitude; it is an extension of personality *beyond* the ego. The ego is the centre, and a complex, of consciousness. It is, however, bound to consciousness and is consequently negative to the unconscious. It does not know what to do about the unconscious and feels it as something totally alien. Individuation consists essentially in recognizing and assimilating the unconscious. Therefore a new centre of personality must come into being, which is not bound to consciousness like the ego but is capable of taking equal account of both consciousness and the unconscious. When we say "must come into being," we are not to be understood as saying that the advent of this new centre can be forced. Normally it simply develops. But the whole psychic process is one of suffering, not an act of will. This new centre Jung calls the "self," and individuation is the way to the self.

The way is long and perilous. It is an encounter with the unconscious, and somehow or other the individual must get into touch with it and accept it. This is not as easy as it sounds. The journey to the unconscious is the "Journey to the Mothers"; and whoever undertakes this journey exposes himself to the perils of the soul. The average European is but scantily prepared for such dangers. He has let himself be persuaded for years that everything to do with the soul is of negligible account, that the soul is something a man hardly needs at all, like the appendix. This being so, he takes no account of all the things that may meet him on the way to the self. There is the danger of possession, that is to say, of the ego's being seized by autonomous complexes. A man may precipitate himself into an archetype and identify himself with it. He may be smitten with such terror of his unconscious that he does not dare to follow the road to an end, and remains stuck. This may have a regressive effect on the personality, i.e. instead of being enlarged it is reduced, because the individual no longer trusts himself. He holds fast to the collective norms and goals, and thus fails to be the very thing he strove for: a personality. In making contact with the unconscious, there is also the danger of the ego's being disintegrated. The psychically sound person will overcome these dangers, albeit with an effort. But there is always the possibility that these encounters and conflicts may bring latent psychoses to the surface. And finally it must never be overlooked that every extension of personality is an extension of consciousness; and making things conscious is no light burden. Consciousness enables us to view the opposites, for instance, in all their sharpness, and this all too easily gives rise to a feeling of inner division. Many things, if not all, are more easily borne when they are unconscious. So that the road that leads to individuation is a wearisome and dangerous one.

The man who wishes to follow the way of individuation successfully must, above all, be loyal to his own fate. There must be no flinching; always he must do what is necessary. Jung expressly proscribes any retreat into the shelter of the Church, even when the conflict with oneself is hard and disagreeable. The Church can, for instance, give us release from guilt through confession. We must not, however, take this way out, but must make ourselves fully conscious of our guilt and its psychic background. The really necessary thing is that we should experience ourselves to the full, get to know our fantasies and what is at the back of them. We must make conscious the contents of all our dreams, reveries, moods; but at the same time always distinguish between contents that can be assimilated to the ego and those that can only be objective to it. For we must realize that psychic factors exist which transcend our own personality and cannot be absorbed into the ego save at the cost of psychic inflation.[48] We should not get engulfed in this. But the conscious experiencing of the psyche makes an enlargement of personality possible, and at the same time we can free the soul from the suggestive power of unconscious images.

Jung mentions some of the experiences to be met with on the way. Thus one meets the shadow, the inferior side of our personality. We must come to terms with it, and, what is more, actively. Individuation cannot be performed at the writing-desk, only in active life. This encounter with the shadow, one's double, Jung calls the "apprentice-piece" in the work of individuation. The "master-piece" is the encounter with the anima—in women, animus. The anima must be experienced and made conscious in the individuation-process so that we may have direct contact with the inner world and the unconscious.

In this way the inferior side of our personality is assimilated to the ego and consciousness is broadened. A broadening of consciousness can also come about by carefully observing everything that reaches us from the inner world. These elements, however, can no longer simply be appended to the ego, because the ego still remains the centre of consciousness and cannot include the unconscious as well. Hence a new centre 'of consciousness has to develop, which Jung calls the *self*. This self is related to consciousness and the unconscious alike and is therefore superior to the ego. Consequently, it acts as a new set of bearings for the man who is following this path. The analysis of the anima and the direct contact with the unconscious which results find expression in an increase of energy for consciousness. The new personality disposes over the energy accruing from the uncon-

[48] *BZIU*, p. 167.

scious, and Jung is not loath to call this personality a "mana-personality."

The birth of a new personality is marked in many cases by the appearance of the *unifying symbol*, which is expressed in various ways. It may show itself in a dream-image. Jung often gets patients to draw these symbols. Very often they are structurally akin to the *mandalas* found in Eastern religions. Such mandalas are symbols of wholeness and indicate that the person in question is on the road to totality and that various contradictory and discrete elements in his personality are on the point of uniting. The mandalas work instrumentally—that is, the patient, by shaping and executing them in his drawings, releases certain psychic processes in himself. Most mandalas contain a fourness, which appears to be something innate in the psyche and thus represents psychic wholeness. It is a pet idea of Jung's that the Christian Trinity is really an imperfect Quaternity. The fourth Person is Satan, who has so far been denied by our rigid adherence to the trinitarian dogma—of which the result is that the wholeness of personality has remained a closed book to Western Christendom. The pact with Mephistopheles in Goethe's *Faust* is symbolic, for Jung, of the spiritual problem of modern man, which is to make a Quaternity of the Trinity, or, in psychological terms, to become whole by recognizing a psychic complex that has so far been denied. Today many persons are struggling for this wholeness.

(As regards the interpretation of the mandalas, about which much has been conjectured, it may be noted that Jung gets his patients to draw them only in order to induce a certain psychic "constellation." The mandala expresses, in empirically accessible terms, a psychic change that we cannot perceive directly. The important thing is not what the mandala palpably shows but the process reflected in it. Mandalas need not necessarily be drawn; they can be expressed in other ways—for instance, in dancing.)

Jung's latest publications are all concerned with the process of individuation. In every religious personality of individual stamp, indications of this kind are discoverable. Also, all historical religions have worked the symbolism of totality into their own particular symbols. We have already mentioned the Christian Trinity. The Cross contains a fourness and is a totality symbol; likewise is the lotus-flower of the Buddhists. Jung also finds traces of religious experiences whose aim is wholeness, and therefore individuation, in all esoteric doctrines. Such traces are to be found in the Catholic Mass, in the teachings of *The Tibetan Book of the Dead*, in *The Secret of the Golden Flower* (which Jung brought out with Richard Wilhelm), in Zen Buddhism, and lastly in alchemy. According to Jung, only a fraction of the last can be regarded as the forerunner of our modern chemistry. The rest is based on the projection of unconscious psychic processes, and alchemistic practices are but the expression of transformations going on unconsciously in the alchemist's psyche. In so far as these processes can be interpreted at all, they are analogous to the process of individuation.

We must, in order to avoid misunderstandings, add that though Jung detects one and the same process of individuation in all religions and cultures, he is far from wanting to put all religions on the same level. The individuation-process displays only formal correspondences in the various religions. But what a man experiences and how he experiences it is different in each case and in each man. That the experiences of one man in one religion should be exactly like those of another in another goes right against the meaning of individuation. Were that so, the one could be taken over ready-made from the other, which is precisely not the case. The important thing is for a man to have the primordial religious experience. The nature of this depends on the nature and psychological make-up of the individual, and the extent to which he gives himself up to his inner fate. It would be to misunderstand Jung very seriously if we assumed that it made no difference whether we take the way of individuation as Orientals or as Occidentals. Jung deals so extensively with the Oriental paths of salvation only because of his view that we Westerners are barbarians in all matters regarding the soul, whereas the Oriental possesses a far greater knowledge of it than we. The Oriental, therefore, is more capable of describing what individuation is about. But the West is ahead of the East in conscious knowledge; hence the Westerner cannot imitate the Oriental, since he starts from different assumptions. Individuation means coming to or becoming oneself, and not imitating foreigners and their experiences. It accords admirably with Jung's views that the well-known student of China, Erwin Rousselle, should relate in one of his lectures (*Eranos-Jahrbuch 1933*) how, when he was taking a course in a Taoist secret society, roughly corresponding to the way of individuation, the Master gave each of them at the end a vade-mecum: a Chinese book to the Chinese, and to him, as a European, the Bible. Since then, he said, the "imitation of Christ" had for him a new and deeper meaning.

Surveying at a glance what Jung has to say about the function of religion, we see that religion always relates to man's wholeness. This is true of the primordial religious experience as it appears in the description we gave of individuation, and also true of the collective religions which elaborate a system of myths, rituals, forms of worship, and traditional dogmas. Jung emphasizes very strongly the compensatory effect of religion, meaning that religion contains and brings out those things which are not realized in our everyday thinking and doing, but which are none the less innate in us. I would refer once again to the compensatory attitude of early Christianity as regards antiquity. We can say, then, that religion gives expression to that which is present but not realized. That is the reason why so many unconscious elements are at work in religion. Even though consciousness may follow different principles, the unconscious functions are still there. The neurotic proves that these can make themselves felt in a highly disquieting manner. It is always possible, however, for them to work themselves out in religion. Then they cease to disturb, and contribute in no small way to personality. A man's behaviour may be influenced very significantly by the archetypes, so much so that they sometimes involve him in courses of action which, from the point of view of making the best of life, must be pronounced meaningless. But when the archetypes are contained in religious symbols, they may be experienced in a meaningful way, so that the archetypes are, in a manner of speaking, exorcized. And even if the myths and symbols harbour all sorts of unconscious elements, these may yet produce a *psychic cosmos instead of a psychic chaos*. All the psychic contents which are touched into life by religion then become related to one another, e.g. the conscious to the unconscious, the spiritual to the natural; all our stirrings and instincts fall into a pattern. The symbols release things in us, create order, and broaden. Psychic functions that might otherwise exert a disturbing influence become positive in their effect. The individual attains to what we described above as *active* experience, which imposes a cosmos on the chaos of his soul.

It is for these reasons that Jung makes the astonishing assertion that religion ministers to psychic hygiene.[49] We have to realize, of course, that Jung is speaking as a psychologist and doctor and not as a theologian. Nor has he any desire to explain away the ultimate core and meaning of religion,[50] any more than the psychologist can explain away art. But on the basis of his experience, he sees himself justified in thinking that a living religion ministers to psychic health. He comes to this conclusion by way of the observation that none of his patients who are over thirty-five years old have yet done with the question of religion. On the other hand, he is seldom visited by people who experience religion as a living thing. In his lecture to the Alsatian Society of Ministers, on "Psychotherapy and the Cure of Souls," he went into the question very deeply and said things of the utmost significance for the theologian. He stated that where the need for a religious orientation is ignored, a neurosis is likely to ensue.[51] In such cases people suddenly become aware of the meaninglessness of their lives, not merely playing with the idea but experiencing it as a veritable inner paralysis. But if symptoms of this kind fail to appear in persons who have a living religion, particularly in the second half of life, then this is a sure indication of some bond between their religious attitude and their mental health.

A proviso must be made here lest the idea be turned into the sort of facile ecclesiastical apologia that would be completely at odds with Jung's intentions. First of all, Jung draws express attention to a fact which is consciously or unconsciously ignored by most theologians—namely,

[49] *PR*, p. 81.   [50] *SPG*, pp. 41.   [51] *Ibid.*, p. 104.

that every attitude can be either genuine or not genuine. A man may be converted to a religion because he has had the experiences formulated in it, and then his conversion is a genuine conversion. But he can also accept this conversion to religion because he needs it to compensate for other things, in which case his conversion is not genuine or is only a figurative conversion. It cannot be seen from the conversion itself whether it is a genuine attitude or not on the part of the individual concerned. A "figurative" conversion may be absolutely correct as to form and content, it may be carried off with the utmost conviction, it may rest on the greatest possible sincerity and yet not be the same thing as genuine conversion. Its function in the individual's personality is quite different from that of genuine religious experience. Like Jaspers in his *Psychologie der Weltanschauungen*, Jung lays great stress on this possibility, that a man's attitude may be merely figurative. In his *Psychology and Religion*, Jung emphasizes that religion, when it really is religion, can never be a substitute.[52] It must be born out of the fullness of life by a man experiencing his life actively and fulfilling all its tasks; then only will he know what he is doing.[53]

When a man's religion is not genuine, it is ineffectual.[54] But an ineffectual religion is no religion at all, because it can have no function in the soul. It can lead at most to the repression of psychic contents, and this is bound to take its revenge. The demand that religion be genuine, that is to say, spiritually connected with certain meaningful experiences, has as its corollary Jung's repudiation of the demand for a dogmatic belief which would entail submission to outside authority, or a *sacrificium intellectus*, no matter how sublime or impressive. For him faith is acceptable only in the sense of *pistis* (trust or confidence),

---

[52] *PR*, pp. 66, 77.   [53] *EJ 1935*, p. 115.   [54] *PR*, p. 58.

but never in the sense that a man must submit to an alleged supermundane truth which cannot be understood by human reason. Religion may not always be reasonable, but it never goes *against* reason, only *beyond* it, because it derives ultimately from the unconscious, where the opposites are close together. Once the contents of a religious faith have been experienced, it will be seen that this is the best possible formulation of that experience, and as such it can be acknowledged; but to demand the acknowledgement of that faith without our having experienced anything to correspond with it is nonsense for Jung. Hence his saying that religion ministers to psychic hygiene should not be twisted into an apologia for religion or used to demand unconditional acknowledgement of any religious system.

Moreover, Jung makes certain demands of religion itself. It must meet psychic facts half-way and *really* give expression to the tendencies and elements existing in the soul. In view of this, Jung's attitude to the existing religions is by no means absolutely positive; he has, indeed, certain reservations to make. Dealing with the archetypes, he says: "An interior spiritual world of which we had no knowledge before is now opening up in front of our eyes and revealing things that stand in the sharpest contrast to all our former ideas. These images are so intense that it is quite understandable why millions of cultivated persons should be taken in by theosophy and anthroposophy. This happens simply because such modern gnostic systems meet the need for expressing and formulating the wordless occurrences going on within ourselves *better* than any of the existing forms of Christianity, not excluding Catholicism. The latter is certainly able to express, far more comprehensively than Protestantism, the facts in question through its dogma or ritual symbolism. But neither in the past nor today has even Catholicism attained anything like the richness of the old pagan symbolism, which is why this symbolism persisted far into Christianity and then gradually went underground, forming currents that have never, from the early Middle Ages to modern times, quite lost their vitality. To a large extent they vanished from the surface; but, changing their form, they are now returning to compensate for the one-sidedness of our conscious mind as orientated today. Our consciousness is so saturated with Christianity, so absolutely moulded by it, that the unconscious counter-position can discover no foothold there, for the simple reason that it is too much the antithesis of our fundamental ideas. The more one-sidedly, absolutely, and rigidly the one position is held, the more aggressive, hostile, and incompatible will the other become, so that at first sight there would seem to be no prospect of reconciling the two. But once consciousness admits at least the relative validity of all human opinion, then the opposition loses something of its irreconcilable character. In the meantime, the conflict casts round for appropriate expression in, for instance, the Oriental religions—Buddhism, Hinduism, Taoism. The syncretism of theosophy meets this need to a very large extent, and this explains its numerous successes." [55]

It is clear from this interesting passage that Jung has certain quite definite reservations to make as regards the existing religions, and that it is not feasible to apply his recognition of religion as a necessary psychic function to every church and confession indiscriminately. It is far from implying a "force them to enter" attitude, or even the defence of an existing religion against any and every form of attack; the only thing that clearly emerges is the

[55] *Ueber die Psychologie des Unbewussten* (Zürich, 1942), p. 140.

question whether any particular religion is the best possible way to realize the potentialities of the soul.

Jung has, of course (to point to this side of his psychology in the present context), gone into the question of the distinction between healthy and pathological psychic life in the field of religion. He affirms that a distinction should be made, and lays great stress on the pathology of religion in his writings. This is a question from which—to its own hurt—theology holds aloof. But as a psychiatrist and psychotherapist Jung has established the existence of many pathological phenomena in religion, and in addition there was the evidence of psychoanalysis to hand. The latter tends to put religion and neurosis on the same level. Jung does not go as far as this, but, on the other hand, one gets a strong impression from his psychology that a man's religious feelings can easily succumb to pathological distortions and aberrations. Despite the fact that the Church and theology sometimes claim to have, as it were, a "corner" in religion, they ignore these things and act as though every manifestation of religious feeling were intrinsically sublime. Hence there is all the more reason for stressing that modern psychology sees things very differently.

Once again we must return to the fact that every religious attitude and every profession of religion may be real or figurative, genuine or non-genuine. A religious creed may be objectively the best possible expression of a man's experiences. It can also be the compensation for quite other things. Psychological law makes it possible for every psychic content to be replaced by another. Thus, a disturbance of sexual life can be the signal for disturbances in a man's relations with his fellows or the world in general. Avarice, a craving for money and possessions may be connected with lack of sexual gratification. This law applies to religion as well. What appears on the surface as a marked religious attitude may be a compensation for things far removed from religion. Underneath a rigid adherence to some religious creed, with respect to which the believer will permit not a jot or a tittle to be altered, there lurks, not an experience of the psychic contents of that creed, but the attempt to erect a barrier against his fear of life. One cannot see from the creed, nor at first sight from the believer himself, whether it rests on genuine or non-genuine religious feeling. Only a deeper knowledge of him can decide. The literature of psychoanalysis offers us a mass of material in this connexion, though the Freudian approach to psychological interpretation is easily schematized and apt to interpret all cases alike. Jung has many more points of view.

But still other phenomena fall to the pathology of religion. When a man experiences elements of the unconscious that he has not assimilated, he may identify himself with them; he gives up his ego in favour of this or that complex and becomes a man possessed. He may perhaps encounter a primordial image—the God-image, for instance—and then we have theomania, where the patient imagines himself to be God. All prophets who, like Antoni Unternährer, believe in unbridled hedonism run similar risks. Or whoever receives from his unconscious revelations and promptings of kinds that do not accord with his conscious thinking may see this as a reason for regarding himself as a being favoured by God. Here, too, Jung's knowledge of the collective unconscious enables us to interpret these things psychologically, since he makes it clear that in certain circumstances we have access to psychic contents which are not of a personal order. The individual has no say whether he shall have these experiences or not. But while one person runs no risk of megalomania, because he makes no attempt to ascribe these contents to his ego, the other may. All the strange instances of possession, and phenomena like glossolalia ("speaking with tongues"), are susceptible of psychological interpretation. They are autonomous complexes which affect the individual's conscious mind from his unconscious.

Further, Jung gives reasons for the peculiar cantankerousness often to be met with in markedly religious persons. In their case the law of compensation is clearly at work, an extreme attitude on the part of the conscious mind evoking its counterpart. There are many pious persons who fail to acknowledge the unconscious and, instead, repress the anima, itself the channel of the unconscious. This is amply avenged, seeing that pious people's moods and fantasies are generally pretty devilish.[56] Among the saints, too, Jung finds persons who carry their religion too far and try to mortify the natural man, with the result that they become split personalities. He tells of a case where he thought that he had really discovered a saint, since he was unable to detect any such split in him. As he (Jung) was about to draw in his horns and modify his judgement on sainthood, the saint's wife came to consult him about her neurosis. The treatment disclosed that the saint had simply let all disturbing elements manifest themselves through his wife, who had to pay with neurosis for the rôle unconsciously assigned to her.[57] Thus, it is always a matter of extremes evoking the appropriate compensation and sometimes leading to a split personality, which may ultimately border on the pathological. Naturally, it is hard to draw the line, and one has to decide in almost every case what is to be described as normal and what morbid. At any rate, the sworn atheist,

[56] PR, p. 135. [57] BZIU, p. 127.

or would-be atheist, also belongs to the category of split men, for Jung is of the opinion that there is no such thing as real irreligion. If consciousness produces no religion, the unconscious will concern itself with it all the more; and the dreams of this type of person are often filled with religious images. The confirmed doubter is, in his unconscious, more religious than he likes to admit, just as the man who wants to abjure all doubt and demonstrate his attitude by violent heresy-hunts is unconsciously all the more wrapped up in his doubt.

We have seen.that theology faces psychology with the question whether there is such a thing as a religious need. Jung recognizes such a need only as the desire to have the facts a man experiences formulated in a religion. For Jung, the basis of religious creeds is not so much a *need* of this sort as *experience*, and this experience is a psychic event which represents certain functions of the psyche as a whole. Religious experience can be defined by saying that it tends towards psychic integration. Religion is the acknowledgement of the things that consciousness fails to realize; or it can go further and bring about an inner unity and wholeness. Thus, religion contributes substantially to a man's total structure, and a living religion is needed for the full development of personality. But owing to its connexion with the psyche, it is also prone to the psyche's dangers, so that religion may well take on pathological forms.

This, in sum, is the answer given by Jung's psychology to the theologian.

The attentive reader will see on closer inspection that there are different kinds of religious persons. Thus, the man who finds what he needs in myths is not religious in the same way as the man who follows the way of individuation. We must therefore discuss this question in another chapter.

MAN AND RELIGION

IT WILL have become apparent from our exposition so far that Jung does not speak of God as an *idea*, but that when he speaks of God at all he means something quite different. God is not thought or contrived, nor is he apprehended and exhausted by our ideas: he is *experienced*. And as long as what a man experiences of God is alive, he is influenced by it. Consequently, Jung prefers to speak of a God-symbol, and he holds that what is true of symbols in general is true also of the God-symbol. He may speak sometimes of a God-image, which is, however, not to be thought of as a metaphorical representation of God, but by the term "image" he means a psychological magnitude. We can reflect on a symbol or psychic image, yet its content can never be formulated exhaustively in terms of ideas—indeed, if it can, the symbol or image has lost its psychic efficacy: it is dead, the perished relic of a psychic state that is no more. Although the God-image must address itself to reason, it must still have something of the irrational at the back of it, something that is pregnant with meaning, that is intuited but not clearly formulated.

Jung associates the God-image with the power of imagination. Imagination is an actualization of the contents of the unconscious, which do not belong to the empirical world and are of an archetypal nature. What happens is that hitherto unconscious fantasies are made conscious through our active participation in them. The fantasies must be taken seriously—this is the active participation— and yet the conscious mind must be there at the same time to realize that the images thrown up by fantasy are not true in themselves but are only expressions of the underlying psychic process. When suicide appears in a dream or fantasy, something "like suicide" is happening in the psyche. Imagination of this sort widens personality, reduces the dominant influence of the unconscious, and brings about a modification of personality itself.[1] In alchemy there were processes of a psychological order that corresponded to imagination. "The concept of *imaginatio* is perhaps the most important key to the understanding of the alchemistic *opus*. The anonymous author of the treatise *De Sulphure* speaks of 'the imaginative faculty of the soul' in that passage where he intends to do just what the ancients had failed to do—that is, put his finger on the secret of the art. The soul, he says, stands in the place of God (*sui locum tenens seu vice Rex est*) and dwells in the life-spirit of the pure blood. The soul functions (*operatur*) in the body, but has the greater part of its function (*operatio*) outside the body. [We may add by way of explanation: in projection.] This peculiarity is divine. For divine wisdom is only in part enclosed within the body of the world; for the greater part it is outside, and imagines far higher things than the body of the world can grasp (*concipere*); and these are outside nature— God's own secrets. The soul is an example of this; it, too, imagines many things of the utmost profundity (*profundissima*) outside the body, as God does. Of course what the soul imagines happens only in the mind; but what God imagines happens in reality. 'The soul, however, has absolute and independent power (*absolutam et separatam potestatem*) to do things that differ (*alia facere*) from those the body can grasp. But it has, when it wishes, the greatest power over the body (*potestatem*

[1] *BZIU*, p. 171.

in corpus), for otherwise our philosophy would be in vain. . . . Thou canst grasp far greater matters, since we have truly opened the doors for thee.' " [2] Since alchemy had little scientific knowledge to offer in the modern sense, but instead, the possibility of projecting psychic contents, it was clearly the expression of psychic processes. Hence imagination is the activation and projection of the same. Alchemistic facts are in reality psychic happenings; and we can indeed say that the alchemists were "fascinated" by the unconscious.[3]

The God-image that men make for themselves in idea is likewise a work of imagination—that is to say, it is not so much a matter of knowledge of some fact external to man as of the expression of a psychic fact, the best possible formulation of some psychic actuality which we have to exteriorize in order to grasp at all.

For the theologian this view of Jung's is a pretty hard nut to crack. It is to be supposed that the theologically minded among our readers will, even if they have had the patience to follow us thus far, advance upon us at this point muttering "psychologism!" as the epithet best fitted to express their critical misgivings. And it does indeed seem as if everything could be resolved into psychological data with Jung and as if the very ground were slipping from under the facts that are the basis of all theological thought and speculation. For the time being it were best to set all such misgivings aside and hold fast to Jung's own axiom that his business is psychology and not theological or philosophical metaphysics. He is investigating religion as a psychologist and starting from psychological assumptions. Just how far his views may or can claim objective truth is a point that we will not attempt to decide for the present.

[2] *EJ 1936*, p. 35.   [3] *Ibid.*, p. 41.

Nevertheless, two things should be noted when Jung speaks of the God-image being moulded by psychic facts: firstly, it does not mean that the God-image is created by human caprice. Jung is absolutely of the opinion that the God-image comes into being on a plane far beyond the caprice of the individual or of any collectivities whatsoever. According to his view of the extent and reality of the psyche, we are dealing here with psychic happenings on the further side of consciousness and personality. Secondly, when Jung calls the God-image a psychic fact, he is not saying that it is "only" psychic. As to why, in the last resort, a God-image should form at all, psychology has as little to say as any other science. The possibility of the soul's being affected by something intensely significant—an event that would then stimulate the formation of a God-image—is one of which Jungian psychology takes full account at the outset. Here, too, we must distinguish between the thing-in-itself and the image of it in the soul, for it is the latter that we have to do with. About the thing-in-itself Jung makes no pronouncement, and there is no fear of falling from the frying-pan of his views, if we acknowledge them, into the fire of Feuerbachian criticism.

Jung's psychology leaves room for the idea that every religion created by the human spirit is man's answer to revelation—indeed, Jung himself evidently reckons with this. Such revelation is clearly beyond the range of human influence: it is experience and grace. Sometimes it is an experience so overpowering as to shatter and slay us. The individual has to receive the revelation through his soul and work on it; hence, if it is to prove effective, it must be translated into psychic terms. Hence, also, revelation is bound up with the psychic functions, and the individual assimilates only so much of the revelation as he can digest psychically (in so far as he is not smitten with madness). Religion is therefore the function through which revelation becomes effective for man. To admit this is not to degrade revelation. It is completely to misunderstand Jung if we accuse him of having no knowledge of revelation. As a psychologist he is not primarily concerned with it; what interests him is the psychic and functional background of religion, and he leaves the question open as to the significance we are to impute to the reality which impinges on man in the process of revelation. The theologian's fear that Jung's psychology may destroy the accepted meaning of revelation rests on a misunderstanding and probably also on the lack of any clear epistemological inquiry into the idea of revelation itself. But we must admit at once that Jung's psychology leaves no room at all for a doctrine of revelation which would satisfy all possible ecclesiastical and theological presumptions in the matter of authority, and these, as we know, are very much in vogue today. Yet we can, not unjustifiably, entertain the opinion that when Jung declines to recognize theological claims of this kind, not he but theology will have to revise its ideas. For such a view of religious authority is not generally recognized even in theological circles, because it cannot be supported by impeccable reasons. The fact, however, that the way to a fuller understanding of revelation even for theologians leads through the soul and not through the apparent certainties is proved by works like St. Augustine's *De Trinitate*, Adolf Schlatter's *Glaubenslehre*, and Hermann Lüdemann's *Dogmatik*.

The close ties between the God-image and the soul may perhaps be recognized even by the Christian theologian when we set foot in what is, for him, neutral territory: the religions outside Christianity. For if we cannot accept the early Christian view that the gods of polytheism are real enough, but are demons or wicked angels, Jungian psychology nevertheless has a plausible explanation to offer. We see from it why the men of earlier times could believe in several gods: they were forces of the unconscious projected into space.[4] Since the intuition of God depends on the mode of consciousness, it will be more or less understandable why men with a not very developed consciousness saw Deity in an altogether different way from that of men possessed of individuality and a wide range of consciousness. The derivation of deities from the forces of nature and from memories of heroes, so common to old-style religious research, leaves a host of unresolved puzzles and questions behind. Moreover, the question is not without relevance for us Christians today. We have only to bear in mind the fact that the whole pagan pantheon has enjoyed the happiest resurrection in the saints of the Catholic Church. And since the Catholic Church was, until four hundred years ago, the sole representative of Christianity, the matter ultimately concerns Protestants as well. If we want, therefore, to make any attempt to understand and interpret religion scientifically, we must address ourselves radically to the problem of what the relationship really is between man and religion, and above all between man and his views of God. If we are now told that the God-image and the images of miscellaneous gods are figures of the unconscious, nothing, it is true, is explained, but at least a relationship has been established.

Jung takes the God-image fundamentally as a *symbol*. He defines the symbol as a union of opposites. Whether this is also the case with the Nature-deities we find in primitive religions is not at first sight obvious. But Jung

[4] *SPG*, p. 325.

points out that the cosmogonic deities and redeemer-gods of primitive religion do in fact possess this characteristic of uniting opposites—in the guise of bisexuality.[5] It is certainly no accident that the union of opposites should appear precisely in the gods who are credited with being world-makers and world-redeemers. The cosmogonic gods are responsible for the discord in the world; they must therefore embrace opposites in themselves. Redemption is conceived largely as the abolition of the discord in man. The need for redemption rests on our experience of inner disunity, of a split in the soul. Redeemer-gods must therefore be able to overcome all opposites. This expresses itself partly in their bisexuality but also in the fact that they are gods who die and rise again. In them death and life are united. Psychologically speaking, this proves their symbolic character.

But something else is connected with this symbolic character—namely, God-images are themselves living things that can die. Jung says the same of the symbol. In every religion the moment will come when the God-image hitherto employed no longer works like a live thing. It may, thanks to the laws of inertia and conservation, which operate very powerfully in the field of religion, persist for a long time as an outward form, but life is not in it. God-images are only valid for a people as a whole when they are alive. On the cessation of their living power, they may continue to be effective for certain persons, while for others they are dead. When a God-image is losing its living power, men feel that their gods are dying: great Pan is dead. The twilight of antiquity was really a vast dying of God.[6] Neither for the individual nor for the community is this moment easy to

[5] Jung-Kerényi: *Introduction to a Science of Mythology*, p. 128; *WSL*, p. 247.

[6] *EJ 1934*, p. 191.

bear. For Nietzsche the statement that God is dead was bound up with a profound spiritual shock that can be noticed in his writings. And the extraordinary religious insatiability that appeared at the end of the classical era, an insatiability that sought peace and salvation everywhere and found it not, gives us some idea of the inner horror of the experience that God is dead. The literature of the war of 1914–18 and its aftermath also bears witness to the same sense of horror, and the spiritual situation following on the last war will doubtless produce similar documents. Subjectively, God's dying is felt as the meaninglessness of existence. People no longer know what they are living for. One of the infallible signs that a God-image is dying is that people begin asking what is the meaning of the God-image or God-symbol.

Whether a God-symbol dies or not depends, as in the case of all symbols, on whether it still corresponds to the state of a man's consciousness. If he has evolved so far that a symbol is no longer the best possible expression for some intuited fact that is of importance to him, then the symbol becomes lifeless. The reasons for this may be very various. The individual may have developed in such a way that a fact which he formerly intuited can now be clearly understood. In that case we are dealing with a broadening of consciousness. But on the other hand, there may be a narrowing of consciousness in an individual or community, so that men are no longer capable of intuiting what is contained in the symbol, which thereupon becomes meaningless. Or a man's experiences may shift to another plane of being, with the result that he no longer has the possibilities of certain earlier experiences at his disposal. The symbols of the Middle Ages, for instance, are derived from a markedly introverted type of mentality—hence they are alien to the predominantly extraverted attitude of today. But whatever the reasons, there is always the possibility of God's dying, and this has serious consequences for the people who experience it.

There is, however, not only the "God-death," the extinction of the God-symbol, but also a renewal of it.[7] God may change with a modification of the God-image.[8] The symbol may in the course of time be replaced by a new one. From the point of view of the psyche this is, indeed, an absolute necessity. In his practice Jung has observed people during the period when a new intuition of God was taking shape in them. He tells us—in the case we have already mentioned, of the patient whom he could help only by continuing the analysis and who had to discover a new meaning for her life *by herself*—how certain contents gradually appeared in her dreams which could not be interpreted at all save as a new God-image. At first, the dreams seemed to indicate the person of the analyst, since they showed him in superhuman proportions and thus had all the appearance of typical transference-dreams so very familiar from the literature of psychoanalysis. But in time Jung became convinced that this could not be the right interpretation, and that a new God-image was clearly being sought in the dreams—that is, a new God-symbol was taking shape.[9] The dreams disclosed a veritable God-seeking, a lusting after God. Gradually a God-image of archaic character was crystallized out, evidently formed in the unconscious.[10] As though in inner harmony with this, the patient developed a new, distinct, and spiritually stable mode of life. Jung gives literary examples of such a renewal of God —above all, in Spitteler.[11]

[7] *PT*, p. 256.
[8] *PR*, p. 151.
[9] *BZIU*, p. 22.
[10] *Ibid.*, p. 24.
[11] *PT*, p. 256.

Here, too, it must not for a moment be supposed that the individual is creating God; it is simply that the supra-personal functions of the psyche are creating the God-image. The genesis of this is not a conscious act of will, as far as the individual is concerned, but, at most, an event which he can actively experience; he cannot determine the course it is to take. A man may recognize or repudiate his God and fight against him, but he cannot ever be rid of him. This can be seen with many converts and atheists. Nietzsche was never able to carry his conflict with Christ to a successful conclusion in the sense of turning to something new and positive.[12] Goethe, on the other hand, never attempted to deviate from his God-image, but strove to deepen it all his life.

From the psychological point of view, therefore, God manifests himself as an autonomous complex of considerable strength and intensity. The God-symbol is ultimately the expression of life's intensity at its highest,[13] and is thus always stronger than consciousness. It can do more than the conscious will can do, for it partakes of the "objective psyche": the material of the unconscious. That is why God is always experienced as power at first and never as idea. But that is also why God is always a moral problem for us, the solution of which is attended by grave difficulties. The God-image is powerful enough to overwhelm the individual ego.[14] Every autonomous complex has its own law, and this is true *a fortiori* of a complex as powerful as the God-image. Ultimately, God is "beyond good and evil." This is implicit in the symbolic character of the God-image itself, since every symbol is the union of opposites; and if moral good is contained in it, so also is moral evil. If the God-image were not a symbol, it would be in-

[12] *EJ 1938*, p. 440.   [13] *PT*, p. 270.   [14] *BZIU*, p. 204.

effectual. It works precisely through its symbolism, but precisely because of this it contains elements that cannot be accommodated to morality. By way of corroboration that God is beyond good and evil Jung cites Meister Eckhart,[15] and also points to Niklaus von der Flüe, who in his visions experienced God as something terrible.[16] That the experience of God has something terrible about it even today is proved for Jung by the universal clamour for leaders.[17] The cry for a leader sounds when men are looking for a *personality*—that is, for a man who has found his own law and is prepared to give effect to it as the determining factor of his life. The man who has become a personality is superior to all others in one respect: he has overcome the panic fear of the psychic and has put the terror of being possessed by it behind him. That is why those who are experiencing the dread sway of supra-personal forces, the "God of terrors" in their very souls, call for a leader. Jung is of the opinion that in experiencing God man partakes of the divine creative power, but that in that case the New Testament saying we have already quoted has all the more relevance: "It is a fearful thing to fall into the hands of the living God."

No doubt many people—not only the theologian but the majority of readers interested in religion—will jib at this expression of Jung's, that God is an autonomous complex, for such an utterance flies in the face of most of our religious teachings. Traditional Christianity in its various confessional forms is accustomed to separate God and the soul no less timidly than categorically. If it is a metaphor for most people nowadays to say that God is in heaven, yet nobody says that God is in the soul. This is just what Jung does say quite logically and, we might

[15] *PT*, p. 343.   [16] *EJ 1934*, p. 186.   [17] *WS*, p. 197.

add, unabashedly. And he says it deliberately, with a view to overcoming once and for all the ancient misunderstanding that everything psychic is "only" psychic and thus somehow inferior as regards the quality of its being. Whatever is psyche or psychic *exists*, and its existence is no whit less significant than physical existence. Jung cites Anselm of Canterbury and Kant in support of his contention that what exists in the soul exists in reality.[18]

It may be that not all our misgivings are assuaged. If we call God an autonomous complex and a symbol whose effects are psychologically measurable, are we not bound to think of God as *relative*? If he is placed in so intimate a relation to the soul, does he not become dependent on the soul? God, we then argue, in so far as he is humanly graspable and psychologically effective, is a God-image and must therefore be a symbol. But symbols are formed in the human psyche. Or again, the whole idea of God evolving and dying seems to point to God's dependence on the soul in the same way that the soul is subject to his influences and experiences them as significant. This would appear to put God's absoluteness in jeopardy and establish his relativity. Jung would say that he recognizes the rightness of these misgivings, but that for his part he would affirm the inference, holding as he does that the doctrine of the relativity of God is a just one. " 'Absolute' means 'detached.' To regard God as absolute is tantamount to placing him outside all human relationships. In that state man cannot influence God, nor God man. A God of this sort would be of no consequence at all. We can in fairness only speak of a God who is relative to man, as man is to God. The Christian idea of God as a 'Father in heaven' puts this

[18] *PT*, pp. 62, 66.

relativity in an exquisite way. Quite apart from the fact that a man can know even less of God than an ant can know of the contents of the British Museum, this urge to regard God as 'absolute' derives solely from the fear that God might become 'psychological.' This would naturally be dangerous. An absolute God on the other hand does not concern us in the least, whereas a 'psychological' God would be real." [19] The result of this separation of God and man is that we have no confidence in man as such, and "all that is left is a miserable, inferior, useless, and sinful little lump called Man."

But Jung is not content to postulate the relativity of God simply because of his own views; he seeks to justify these by historical and psychological references. He casts about him for religious-minded people who, purely from their own religious experience, have put forward a similar view of God in which he is relative to the human soul. He finds such a view in the writings of the German mystics Meister Eckhart and Angelus Silesius.

In Meister Eckhart Jung finds above all else an *appreciation* in the value of the soul which is in keeping with his own psychological views. Jung quotes Eckhart as saying: "For man is truly God, and God truly man." [20] "He, on the contrary, for whom God is not an inward possession, but who must fetch all God for himself from outside in this thing or in that, wherein he will then seek Him unsufficingly through certain works, persons, or places: such a man has Him not, and then something may easily befall to trouble him. And not merely evil company will then trouble him, but also the good; not merely the street, but also the church; not merely evil words and works, but the good likewise. For the

[19] *BZlU*, p. 198 n.   [20] *PT*, p. 343.

stumbling-block lies in himself: God has not yet become world for him. Were God that for him, he would feel himself safe and at ease in all places and among all people: always he would have God." [21] Here Jung sees the proof of his contention that for Meister Eckhart God was a psychological quantity.

"Yet again you must understand the soul to be the Kingdom of God. For the soul is of like nature with the Godhead. Therefore all that is said here of the Kingdom of God, so far as God Himself is this Kingdom, can truly be said of the soul. All things came to pass through Him, says St. John. This is to be understood of the soul, for the soul is all things. It is so, because it is an image of God. But as such it is also the Kingdom of God. So deeply, says one master, is God in the soul that His whole Godliness rests upon it. That God is in the soul is a higher condition than that the soul is in God; for the soul is not yet blessed from being in God, but blessed indeed is the soul which God inhabits. Be certain of this: God is Himself blessed in the soul!" [22] By God's being in the soul Meister Eckhart means the soul's creativeness. The "blessed" condition is therefore a creative condition. For this reason Meister Eckhart can say: "When people ask me, 'Why do we pray, why do we fast, why do we all good works, why are we baptized, why is God become man?' I make answer, 'We do thus that God may be born in the soul and the soul again in God. Therefore was the Holy Script written. Therefore did God create the whole world: that God might be born in the soul and the soul again in God. The inmost nature of all grain means the wheat, of all metal, gold, and of all birth, man!' " [23]

[21] *Ibid.*, p. 344.
[22] *Ibid.*, p. 345. [The German contains an untranslatable play on words: "*Gott ist selber selig in der Seele.*"—TRANS.]   [23] *Ibid.*, p. 351.

Here Meister Eckhart is clearly establishing God's undoubted dependence on the soul. God is born in the soul, and Eckhart speaks of God's birth as a continuous process. At the same time, according to Jung, this process is for the most part unconscious and can only be expressed in metaphorical language. For Meister Eckhart "the soul, through her creatureliness, first made God, so that before the soul was made a created thing there was no God. But a little while and I declared: 'That God is God, thereof am I a cause!' God's being is of the soul, but His Godhead is of Himself. God, too, comes to pass and passes away [literally: becomes and unbecomes]. Because all creatures declare God, God comes to pass. . . . While yet I stood in the ground, in the depths, in the flow and fount of Godhead, no man questioned me whither I went and what I did: there was none there to question. Only when I flowed out did all creatures declare God. . . . And why do they not declare the Godhead? All in the Godhead is one, and of this there is nothing to be said. God alone works, but the Godhead works not; there is no work for it to do and no working in it. Never did it contemplate anything of work. God and Godhead are as different as doing and not-doing. . . . When I again come home into God there is no more doing in me, and this my [striving to] break through [into God] is a far nobler thing than my first flowing out [from God]. I, the One, bring all creatures out of their mind into my mind, that they may become one in me. But when I go back into the ground, into the depths, into the flow and fount of Godhead, none will ask me whence I have come or whither I go. None will have missed me. God passes away." [24]

We see from this that Meister Eckhart distinguishes

[24] *Ibid.*, p. 355.

151

between God and Godhead: Godhead is Total Reality, which neither knows nor possesses itself, while God is a "working" (function) of the soul, the soul in its turn being a working or function of the Godhead.

In this connection Jung also quotes the following verses from Angelus Silesius: [25]

I know that without me
God can no moment live;
Were I to die, then He
No longer could survive.

I am as great as God,
And He is small like me;
He cannot be above
Nor I below Him be.

In me God is a fire
And I in Him its glow;
In common is our life,
Apart we cannot grow.

He is God and man to me,
To Him I am both indeed;
His thirst I satisfy,
He helps me in my need.

God is such as He is,
I am what I must be;
If you know one, in truth
You know both Him and me.

I am the vine, which He
Doth plant and cherish most;
The fruit which grows from me
Is God, the Holy Ghost.

[25] Ibid., p. 359.

So that in Angelus Silesius too, if in less elaborate form, we meet with the doctrine of God's dependence on man. Jung is quite right in stating that the very oddity of this doctrine, which departs so strongly from everything that the West has taught hitherto, forbids us to take it simply as an empty speculation. It is knowledge acquired by men who have learned how to listen to their inmost souls and to experience what comes from the inner side of life. Jung feels himself supported accordingly, and thinks that his views cannot therefore be set aside as mere aberrations but deserve serious attention. The doctrine of the relativity of God ultimately rests on an experience which comes as the result of a certain historical and spiritual constellation. Jung believes that the basic conditions for a renewed approach to these ideas are present today, since they lie in the modern man's field of knowledge—above all, in his knowledge of the nature and meaning of the psyche. In this respect Jung is supported by other investigators. For even those who cannot follow all the details of Jung's psychology can see from the Reformers or from a person like St. Augustine that some connexion must exist between an individual's psychic structure and his idea of God. The relation between soul and God-image is thus ascertainable, and the doctrine of the relativity of God tries to define this relationship more closely.

It may appear strange that the psychologist Jung should absorb such a doctrine into his scientific theories. But that he really is striking a chord in the soul of modern man is proved by the fact that a poet like Rainer Maria Rilke, who was, in his way, deeply interested in religion and the soul, also asserts the relativity of God in his *Stundenbuch*. Jung nowhere takes any account of Rilke, but evidently the psychologist and the poet have stumbled on psychic facts that cannot yet be assessed in their true significance. It is surely more than coincidence that two such utterly different people, each starting from a different point and following a different road, should meet in their vision of God.

Jung is fully aware that this doctrine is not easy to accept, for ultimately it is the sort of knowledge that harbours great perils for mankind. The theologian, above all, will approach it with misgivings that are not without some justification. Does not this doctrine, he will ask, lead to a deification of man, and is not the end-result of a deification of man limitless pride, of the kind we know all too well in certain cranky founders of sects? These misgivings are right: it may indeed happen, but it need not inevitably happen. In fact, the moment God is related to the soul in this way, he becomes dangerous. "It is a fearful thing to fall into the hands of the living God." This is the literal truth, and Jung's psychology has nothing to add to it save that life is probably always dangerous for anybody who wants to live it wholly and that in this world all of us have obviously, albeit for reasons we know nothing of, to deal with dangerous things. All poisons are dangerous, yet without poisons there would be no medicines. Poverty and riches are equally dangerous for the soul, yet all men must be either rich or poor.

For the theologian, perhaps, the last word has not been said nor the last suspicion set at rest. In order to form a clear picture of Jung's teachings in all their implications, he could not do better than to refer to Meister Eckhart's distinction between God and Godhead. Jung would urge such a reference to Eckhart, since he himself cites him and makes copious use of the views of the mystics. This distinction between God and Godhead explains Godhead as the Absolute, which is beyond the soul in every sense and thus not to be recognized or grasped by man as such. God, however, is that part or function of Godhead which is in touch with us and affects us and which we are therefore able to grasp as real. The situation is analogous in Jung. When he as a psychologist speaks of God or the God-image (the two terms are interchangeable), he means the reality that affects us and is thus far experienceable. But what the final cause is, or the final meaning, of the fact that we experience a God-image at all, what is behind the effect it has upon us, about this he will make no pronouncement as a psychologist. He leaves room for the possibility that there is some kind of reality at the back of it, a reality to which the term "Absolute" must undoubtedly be given but about which he can say nothing more within the framework of his science, because we stand here at the limits of all possible science. This reality which affects us and releases the God-image in us and makes it a psychologically definable function can be taken as the creative power innate in all being and all life—indeed, this way of taking it is the only possible one.

The fundamental difference between Jung and the majority of theologians today lies not so much in these individual points which admit of discussion as in the fact that Jung reckons with the possibility and reality of a revelation that can be experienced *now*, whereas theology inclines to regard revelation as unique and finished. In theory Catholicism reckons with continued revelation, but in practice it recognizes as revelation only what agrees in all particulars with the earlier one, which has received ecclesiastical approbation. This is tantamount to prescribing the ingredients of revelation beforehand and judging it by a canon derived from the past. Many branches of Protestantism recognize only a single unique revelation—namely, that recorded in the Scriptures—and refuse to acknowledge any further revelations at present. Other branches of Protestant theology, the so-called free ones, may do so, but they are in a minority. This is a position which Jung takes up and defends with all possible emphasis. The question whether we should reckon with a unique or a continued revelation cannot be decided scientifically. It is one of those questions which the individual must answer out of his own experience and attitude to life. In any theological discussion of Jung's views, this fact must be borne in mind.

Jung puts it beyond all possible doubt that the experience of God, which brings God home to us as a living quantity and not merely as an object of faith in the sense that we acknowledge or subordinate ourselves to a traditional dogma, is an extremely dangerous and terrible thing. Psychically, it claims the whole man, and it is a fatality which may land him in greater spiritual distress and disaster than many of the purely outward circumstances we so dramatically call "fate." When Niklaus von der Flüe left his family and became a hermit, he went because the vision of God that came upon him was so heavy with meaning that he was forced to examine his heart in the most radical way. Just as an artist can work out his vision only by exteriorizing it in a work of art, so Niklaus von der Flüe had to bend to his vision and work it out in himself. When the experience of God is a real living thing, it touches us to the quick, and time and strength are needed in order to come to terms with it. In moments like these we feel the perils and ambiguities of life not only in the surrounding world, not only in our own bodies, but in our very souls; then they are as close to us as they possibly can be, are as dangerous and terrible as they possibly can be, and in certain circumstances are also as rapturous as they possibly can be.

The fact that the God-image operates in this way—which we have instanced in some detail in order to make what follows intelligible—is really at the bottom of man's whole attitude to religion. Because the living experience of God is anything but harmless and easy to master, man has never adopted a single, unambiguous attitude to religious experiences of this kind. On the contrary, the possible attitudes are very numerous, and to these Jung has devoted a good part of his psychological research.

Since religious experience is so devastating in its effects, it comes only to the few. It is fate in a two-fold sense: Firstly, those who have this living experience of God are transformed by it, and the whole course of their lives is changed. Secondly, it is a form of passion or suffering that simply comes over them unawares—something they cannot influence or compel. Or rather, to put it more carefully: they cannot compel it without considerably remoulding their lives, and this only serves to keep their souls "swept and garnished" for the experience if it wants to come, but force it to come they cannot. On the other hand, since psychic facts are always striving for the sort of expression that religion offers, it is possible for a man to borrow from those who have had a personal experience of God *their* God-image and their formulation of this experience. If one is fortunate enough to meet such a person, one becomes his *disciple.* One has then found a solution but is, at the same time, exempt from a religious experience of one's own with all its perils and hazards. There is no reason why one should take on oneself all the difficulties that are the portion of a real prophet. Just how difficult a prophet's life may be can be seen, for instance, in Jeremiah. Since not all of us could stand the strain, there is this more comfortable solution. Naturally, it depends on the accident of meeting a person who has had a genuine religious experience, and such individuals are rare—and perhaps not so easy to recognize. The history of religion, Christianity included, has clearly shown that there are true and false prophets and that the two species cannot always be marked off from one another, at least during their lifetimes. It is not for nothing that the Catholic Church defers beatification for so long. The way of discipleship is thus not entirely without its risks. The Bible, too, advisedly warns against false prophets—which does not prevent upstart prophets from finding disciples even now, irrespective of whether they be true or false. Discipleship is in fact an archetypal attitude—something that is always occurring.

But because it depends on the merest accident and because of its inevitable uncertainty, this solution cannot be regarded as final. Of far greater significance is another substitute for personal experience of God, and that is the Church.

Jung expressly distinguishes between Church and religion. A man who is in the Church does not experience living religion, but puts himself under the influence of what the Church has to offer—dogma, worship, the Church as institution. All religions lead in time to the formation of churches and dogmas, but for Jung real religious experience does not coincide with worship and dogma. On the contrary: the Church interposes itself between the individual and the unconscious,[26] and since

[26] *Ibid.*, p. 76.

the latter is the seat of religious experience, Jung comes to the conclusion, which must seem odd at first, that the Church interposes itself between man and religious experience, or rather, the primordial religious experience. This would appear to be a stringent criticism of the practical value of the Church, and consequently many critics of Jung's book *Psychology and Religion* were amazed and irritated when Jung started by declaring that the effect of the Church was to obstruct the growth of any real and personal religion, and then went off for pages on end into what was almost a paean of praise for the Church—and the Catholic Church at that.

The contradiction, however, is a surface one only. For it is inevitable that, owing to the strangeness and ambiguity of primordial religious experience, this should remain beyond the ken of most people, indeed the great majority, and that they should content themselves with the sort of religion which has taken on fixed forms of dogma and worship and therefore no longer serves to establish contact with the unconscious. Hence Jung approves the Church—only, he would call what the "believer" experiences not a "religion" but a "creed." At the same time, Jung regards it as an absolute psychic necessity for many persons that they should have a "creed" of this kind. For it is only when a man has a creed through which he can express the contents of his unconscious that he is capable of cultural work.

In his *Psychology and Religion*, Jung extols dogma as being more valuable than any scientific theory in this respect. "Taken in itself, any scientific theory, no matter how subtle it may be, is of less value, I should say, from the point of view of psychological truth, than religious dogma, for the simple reason that a theory is necessarily abstract and exclusively rational whereas dogma always expresses an irrational whole in its images. This guarantees a far better rendering of an irrational fact like the psyche. Moreover, dogma owes its continued existence and its form firstly to the so-called 'revealed' or immediate experiences of 'gnosis'—for instance, the God-man, the Cross, the Virgin Birth, the Immaculate Conception, the Trinity, etc.—and secondly to the ceaseless collaboration of many minds over many centuries. It may not be altogether clear why I call certain dogmas 'immediate' experiences, since in itself a dogma is the very thing that precludes 'immediate' experience. Nevertheless, the Christian images I have mentioned are not peculiar to Christianity alone (though in Christianity they have undergone a development and intensification of meaning not to be found in any other religion). We meet them no less in the pagan religions, and apart from that they can reappear spontaneously in all sorts of variations as psychic phenomena, just as, in the dim past, they were born of visions, dreams, and trances. Ideas like these are never invented. They came into being before mankind had learned to use the mind purposively. Before men had learned how to produce thoughts, thoughts came to them. They did not think, but they took note of their mental functions. Dogma is like a dream, reflecting the spontaneous and autonomous activity of the objective psyche, the unconscious. Such an expression of the unconscious is a much more effective means of defence against further immediate experiences than any scientific theory. The theory will inevitably neglect the emotional values of the experience. Dogma, on the other hand, is extremely eloquent in just this respect. A scientific theory is soon overtaken by another; dogma endures for centuries. The figure of the sorrowing God-man must be at least five thousand years old, and the Trinity is probably even older." [27]

The beauty of dogma lies in its supra-personal quality, and in this it expresses all the things the individual intuits or experiences. That is why Jung ends his book with words to the effect that unthinking fools will attack Christian dogma and its symbolism, but not lovers of the soul.

At the same time we must be clear in our own minds that, for Jung, Christianity in its ecclesiastical form (be it noted: in its *ecclesiastical* form) is best represented by the Catholic Church. He regards this as historically proved. The functions of Christianity were taken over by the Catholic Church at the outset. It was necessary for Christianity to create a church, and it is no accident that this church became the Catholic Church. At all periods of its history the Catholic Church has understood how to exercise a paramount influence on mankind.

Jung calls it the greatest objectification of psychic symbols the West has ever known, and is of the opinion that the existence of the Catholic Church is an absolute necessity for many people. It gives them the means of getting into *indirect* touch with the unconscious, and it —and it alone—can give them these means. Any other way would be too difficult and dangerous for their psyches, and they find the optimum psychic conditions for this contact only within the fold of the Catholic Church. The very indirectness of the contact protects them from all the incalculable consequences that flow from a direct encounter with the unconscious.[28] The Church absorbs the archetypes, thereby creating a psychic cosmos instead of psychic chaos.[29] It also has the

[27] *PR*, p. 84 f.   [28] *EJ 1934*, p. 188.   [29] *SPG*, p. 170.

power to exorcize that shimmering, protean, exasperating soul-image, the anima. In Catholic symbolism we find the whole inventory of the unconscious. Everything is contained in it in an orderly manner, and the man who places himself under the influence of this symbolism avoids all further conflict with the unconscious.[30] The "mystical body" of the Church takes full account of the lack of psychic unity.[31] The relevant passage showing the influence which the organization of the psyche has on the formation of religious doctrines runs as follows: "In the manifold phenomenology of the 'child' [i.e. the mythical figure of the 'Divine Child'], we have to distinguish between the *unity* and *plurality* of its respective manifestations. Where, for instance, numerous homunculi, dwarfs, boys, etc. appear, having no individual characteristics at all, there is the probability of a *dissociation*. . . . If the plurality occurs in normal people, then it is a case of the representation of an as yet incomplete synthesis of personality. The personality (viz. the 'self') is still in the *plural stage*, i.e. an ego may be present, but it cannot experience its wholeness within the framework of its own personality, only within the community of the family, tribe, or nation; it is still in the stage of unconscious identification with the plurality of the group. The Church takes due account of this widespread condition in her doctrine of the *Corpus Mysticum*, of which the individual is by nature a member." [32]

In the Catholic Mass we have a representation of the inner change which corresponds to the individual's experience of individuation. The Catholic service tries to realize the union of opposites in a Christian form.[33]

[30] *UES*, p. 99.   [32] *Ibid.*, p. 103.   [33] *PT*, p. 311.
[31] Jung-Kerényi: *Introduction to a Science of Mythology*, p. 116.

Catholicism has also tried consciously to solve this problem by the doctrine of probabilism. Probabilism in moral questions consists in the principle of letting oneself be guided not by one's conscience but by what is probably right, i.e. recommended by some representative authority or doctrine. Catholic moral theology countenances, in short, the following view: in cases not forbidden outright by moral law, it is permissible to hold a sufficiently probable opinion, even when the opposite opinion may be more probable. "Probable" means an opinion supported either by external reasons (the authority of one eminent theologian or more) or by "reasons of the heart." [34] Probabilism is generally described as an outgrowth of the confessional, and one which makes for ethical muddle-headedness. It has even been called "the art of turning conscience into a probability calculus," which is universally practised wherever human egotism and passions influence action. But accusations such as these are repudiated even by the Protestant exponents of probabilism. In his last publication, *Psychology and Alchemy*, Jung sees in probabilism rather the conscious attempt to offer a practical solution of the problem of opposites. He also regards the Pope-symbol as far more effective psychologically than the Protestant predilection for the authority of the Bible. Both historically and psychologically, therefore, he finds

[34] [As our author's formulation of this doctrine is somewhat elliptical, I give two definitions from *The Century Dictionary:* a) "The doctrine that when there are two probable opinions, each resting on apparent reason, one in favour of and the other opposed to one's inclination." b) "When a doubt arises as to the binding force of some divine or human precept in any given case, it is permissible to abandon the opinion in favour of obedience to the law—technically known as 'safe' (*tuta*) opinion—for that which favours non-compliance, provided this laxer opinion be 'probable.' And by 'probable' is meant any judgement or opinion based on some reasonable grounds, though with some doubt that the opposite view is perhaps the true one."—TRANS.]

the best possible realization of the church-principle as such in the Catholic Church.

Jung comes to the same conclusion on comparing Catholicism with other psychological methods of solving the problem of coming to terms with the soul. Buddhism, too, tries to help man to face his unconscious by training his attention on the self. But Catholicism understood how to do one thing which this method failed to do: it objectifies the whole symbolism of the unconscious, i.e. places it outside the individual. In this way, always provided that the symbols of Catholic dogma and ritual are still effective for him, he is spared any conflict with his psyche, and thus he has no need of any psychology. The whole thing is projected, objectified, and consequently "exorcized" (bound by an oath). The Mass shows how subtle are the psychological techniques that the Catholic Church has at its disposal. In the Mass, Christ is shown as a living quantity and reality—he in whom God's sacrifice is consummated over and over again and who can thus offer us salvation anew every day through the transubstantiation.[35] The Mass represents, in objective form, God become man and man become God. Psychologically, too, the exercises of Ignatius Loyola are extremely shrewd. In other religions there are exercises—yoga, for instance. But whereas yoga stimulates the *personal* production of symbols and thus brings the practitioner into the closest possible contact with the unconscious, the Catholic exercises replace the personal production of symbols by carefully chosen elements, so that the individual is insulated against the perils of the soul—but also, be it noted, against its beneficent influences. He gets the experience of Catholic dogma, but not of his own psyche.[36]

[35] *EJ 1936*, p. 52.   [36] *EJ 1935*, p. 66; *Bardo Thödol*, p. 32.

Jung is fully aware that the Catholic Church is not the sole representative of Christianity. We have already pointed out how fond Jung is of substantiating certain of his views on dogma by unofficial currents of opinion, some of them esoteric and condemned by the Church, as for instance in the matter of whether it would not have been better for Christian symbolism to have developed a Quaternity instead of a Trinity. He knows that there are other, underground forms of Christianity besides the official Catholic one. These tendencies he calls "gnostic," and he regards them as extending from early Christian gnosticism right up to alchemy and all its ramifications. He explains the birth of an underground gnosticism alongside the official Christianity of Catholicism like this: the Church was unable to absorb into its dogma and ritual certain portions of classical mythology which were too naturalistic, and had therefore to repudiate them.[37] This process can be seen historically in the suppression of gnosticism by the nascent Catholic Church. Traditional Christianity, therefore, and particularly Catholicism, failed to make man whole. The Christian man, in so far as he remains inside the Church and its traditional doctrines at all, is not "whole," but fragmentary. The Church was never able to extirpate gnosticism completely; it continued despite all suppression and persecution. From gnosticism the line runs to alchemy and thence to the Faust-figure. But since the rejected portion of mythology still represented part of the unconscious psyche, the matter could not be wished away by force. The fragment of psyche that asserted itself in mythology existed, regardless of what councils and Popes might decide. The thing that the Church rejected and condemned in gnosticism was

[37] *PR*, p. 175.

nature—the nature in the unconscious. The Church was bound to suppress nature in order to build up a culture. Otherwise, Christian culture could not have advanced beyond that reached by antiquity, which paid too much attention to nature. Nevertheless, nature and the unconscious continued to assert themselves in a few extraordinary spirits, such as Paracelsus. That is why Jung says of him that he was at once Christian and primitive pagan.[38] Christian symbolism was not redemptive for him, because he intuited that portion of the psyche which Catholicism had no wish to know. The Christ of the Church bears no likeness to the "whole" man.[39] Reacting against this, Paracelsus turned to alchemy and the nature-containing symbolism handed down from of old by the Gnostics. He had to turn to them because they contained that portion of the psyche which he intuited in himself and which the traditional symbolism of the Church either ignored or suppressed. Consequently, he could not simply "believe," i.e. submit to the Church and live in it; he had to look for his own experience.

Until modern times this problem of the inadequacy of Christian dogma did not become acute, nor is it so for many people today. Jung is of the opinion that there are still numerous persons who find a satisfactory solution to their spiritual troubles in the Church. He speaks of *born Catholics;* and when, for instance, somebody comes to consult him and shows that the traditional Christian symbolism of the Church is still operative in his case, Jung sends him back to the Church without compunction, bidding him make use of its psychological techniques. He also says that it is a quite satisfactory conclusion to a course of psychotherapeutic treatment

[38] *Paracelsica*, p. 177.   [39] *Ibid.*, p. 149.

when a patient finds his way back to the symbolism of the Church. For it is pointless to detach a man from the Church if there is no inner need for it. Any other way of healing would be much more difficult and dangerous for him. That is why Jung, as a "lover of the soul," does not attack Christian dogma and symbolism; and if he can facilitate a man's return to the fold he sees this as the goal of his medical treatment.

But clearly and unequivocally as Jung lays this down in his writings, there is another discovery which is equally clear and unequivocal for him—namely, that there are people today for whom a return to the Church is no longer possible, and to these people Jung gives the name "Protestants."

The "Protestant" person, in the Jungian sense, is not simply the representative of a second Christian confession running alongside Catholicism—he is, religiously and spiritually, in a fundamentally different situation. He is not to be identified with the members of the Reformed and Protestant Churches. Among these there are "Protestants" in Jung's sense and many who are on the verge of becoming so. But there are also "Protestants" in communities outside the Church and among those who still have relations of some sort with Christianity but who can discover no inner affinity between themselves and any religious community. In the Reformed Churches, however, there are not only Protestants in Jung's sense but also many whose spiritual home is really the Catholic Church. The Catholic tendencies that are always cropping up in certain denominations of Protestantism prove that there are still a great many people in the Protestant fold who are moved by inclinations for which the Catholic Church has devised the most perfect expression.

Jung's division between his "Protestants" and the members of the Protestant Churches has its good reasons, and no wonder. For nearly one and a half millennia Christians have with but few exceptions lived in the Catholic fold, and the passage of time since the Reformation is, from the point of view of the history of the human soul, relatively short. If, then, the forces which have held men so long to Catholicism still make themselves felt in those who no longer confess the Catholic faith, that is hardly surprising. Further, not every man can choose of his own accord the ecclesiastical community to which he wants to belong; most of us are born into one. Therefore, granted that the spiritual impulses which bring a man to the brink of Catholicism are strongly alive in him, he will always try to give a Catholic twist to the community in which he lives. Hence, though there may be genuine Protestants in the Protestant Churches, they are not the only people in them. In the Catholic Church one seldom finds "Protestants" in the Jungian sense, seeing that, for both internal and external reasons, they would have to quit it. A decision of this kind is not demanded by the Reformed Churches of the genuine Protestant, nor of the man who has a secret longing for Catholicism and the spiritual shelter it affords.

From the psychological point of view Jung regards the Reformation as a turning-point of the profoundest significance—even more profound, perhaps, than it appears to the historian. The Reformation did not, says Jung, simply modify this or that detail in the Catholic system, nor did it merely induce certain changes in dogma, symbolism, worship, and the structure of the Church: it brought about a completely new psychic attitude. We have seen that the Catholic Church is, in

Jung's words, the greatest objectification of religious symbols that the West has known. What the Reformation did was to undertake nothing less than a colossal demolition of this objectification. All the psychic contents which the religious symbolism of the Catholic Church had projected into the surrounding world were *taken back* into the psyche.[40] The old symbols accordingly lost their strength and effectiveness and had to be replaced by new ones. But, projection having ceased, man's relation to God became totally different. The sign that the old Catholic symbolism was no longer valid was the outbreak of iconoclasm.[41] The Reformation was always in essence iconoclasm, and it has gone on being iconoclastic right up to the present. To this somewhat piquant statement of Jung's one may, of course, raise the historical objection that Luther did not countenance iconoclasm—which was the reason why he broke with Karlstadt. But we must not take Jung's interpretation too literally. All he means to say is that the Reformation initiated the demolition of traditional Christian symbolism in worship, dogma, and the Church generally. And in this he is quite right. One has only to enter a modern Reformed church to be struck by its soberness and bleakness. Protestantism has abolished images so thoroughly that even Protestants are sometimes depressed by the austerity of their churches. Then think of the demolition of dogma that has been going on ever since the Reformation and is being continued today in neo-Protestantism. From the psychological point of view the Protestant Churches and their affiliated sects are afflicted with an unparalleled *dearth of imagery* both with regard to the use of art and in dogma itself, so that the Reformation must necessarily appear as sheer icon-

[40] *PT*, p. 360. [41] *EJ 1934*, p. 189.

oclasm no matter whether it be pursued with violence or with the subtler aid of scientific criticism.

The change that the Reformation ushered in as regards Catholic symbolism did not lie within the power of the individual to control. The dearth of imagery rested on the fact that the images and symbols had nothing more to say to great numbers of men. For those who had detached themselves from the Catholic Church the symbols were already dead. Contemplating them, these people discovered that they had no ideas whatever about them, that they were powerless to think of anything, that they experienced nothing, that they saw in them only dead forms and dead matter of no emotional significance. Behind this apparently inexplicable fact lay another, of crucial importance historically: namely, that from a certain point in time it was quite impossible for many people to go on projecting psychic contents into the surrounding world. Catholicism virtually consisted in this projection, which turned the various images and institutions into meaningful symbols. Hence the cessation of projection meant the inhibiting of that spiritual attitude so characteristic of the genuine Catholic. Just why all possibility of projection should have ceased is something of which we do not know the ultimate reasons even today. It hinges on some kind of inner change which, like many scientific facts, we can verify but not explain.

Jung points out that this psychic change did not begin all of a sudden with the Reformation but had started much earlier: in German mysticism—above all, with Meister Eckhart. It was he who took the decisive step, since, with his doctrine of "the little spark of the soul," he withdrew God from the surrounding world and established him in the soul of man. By so doing he switched the projection of the God-symbol away from the Catholic Church. If God dwells in the soul, the Church, together with its hierarchy, ritual, and dogma, automatically loses all divine authority and its supernatural aura. Naturally enough, Eckhart did not simply *invent* his doctrine as a result of inquisitive speculation; he was only voicing what he had experienced. Indeed, we must assume that other people had experienced the same thing; that this change in man's experience and intuition of God was a change in the collective psyche. A new time was coming. The symbol disintegrated from within, in the soul. Unconscious changes were at work which the individual man did not notice and could not have understood. Outwardly, on the surface, little was different. But the Catholic Church had a fine nose for these things and knew that Meister Eckhart was not a Christian in the orthodox Catholic sense. That is why it tried him for heresy—a procedure that was not at all suited to put a brake on the transformation that was going on and make it go backwards. Nothing could now be done about it, for in Meister Eckhart's inversion of man's view of God the real cause was a life-process in the soul itself, which could no more be put into reverse than any other living process.

At all events, the Church seems to have felt something of this change. The existence of a court of inquisition at the time of Meister Eckhart only proves that scepticism had already attained considerable proportions and that the nerve-centre of the Church was fully alive to it. The Church was reckoning with scepticism at that time. Its authority was beyond question only so long as the symbols were living things and thus had absolute validity; so long, therefore, as the Church could attract the contents of the unconscious and bind them to the world of Christian symbols. Meister Eckhart suddenly made it possible for the individual to have direct access to God through his own soul. Even if he himself failed to draw all the conclusions, a time was bound to come when somebody would get up and say what was only too logical: God does not dwell in the Church or in its images and symbols, and therefore we have no further need of it as a mediator. The world of images is meaningless.

This was the conclusion the Reformers drew. Hence Jung sees the Reformation as the direct continuation of German mysticism—a connection which is also grasped by the historian, though he may take other causes into account such as economic, political, and philosophical factors. It was not for nothing that Luther buried himself in the *Theologia Germanica*. The Reformation, however, did not go forward without check. This is shown by the struggle over the Communion between Luther and Zwingli. For Luther the Communion still had a sacramental, symbolical meaning, so that though he abandoned the doctrine of transubstantiation, he accepted that of consubstantiation instead. Catholicism declared that the Communion elements, the bread and the wine, were actually transformed into the flesh and blood of Christ. Luther said that though these substances remained bread and wine, yet, for the believer, the body and blood of Christ were invisibly present at the consummation of the Communion. Psychologically speaking, he was still projecting certain psychic elements of faith, as he experienced it, into the substance. Zwingli took the Communion as a mere sign that the passion and death of Christ are remembered, and said that in reality it was a matter of bread and wine alone. Thus, in him the projection had ceased altogether. From the historical point of view, i.e. as regards the origins of the Christian sacraments, Luther was more in the right, for the Communion was a symbol and not just a sign. But from the point of view of Protestant principle Zwingli was the more consistent, and the history of dogma and sacrament has proved Zwingli right, since Protestantism no longer has any real knowledge of what a symbol is, having taken the projection of religious experience back into the psyche.

This psychological and historical crisis threw up many thorny problems for the Reformers and their successors —above all, the question of where authority was now to be found in religious matters. Catholicism had a ready answer since, by superimposing the God-image on the hierarchical structure of the Church, it invested the Pope as supreme head with absolute authority in all his decisions. The dogma of the infallibility of the Pope is rooted in the nature of Catholicism. It does not need to be proved —the projection of such significant psychic contents into the Church is itself sufficient reason for a dogma of that kind. By taking back the projection the Reformation deprived the Church of its authority, but could not in the circumstances remain without authority. So it made its authority the Bible, despite the fact that people well knew that Luther had treated some of the books of the Bible very cavalierly and that the Bible was not suited to be an absolute authority. Hence the authority the Bible exercised was not authentic. It had to be interpreted, and Christians have never been agreed on the right interpretation of the Bible, not even the Reformers themselves, as their disputations and the resulting dissensions amply show. After the Reformation Protestantism went further in this direction. The perpetual struggle to demonstrate that the Bible is *the* authority in Protestant Christianity has proved unsuccessful, despite all the diligence and energy expended. To speak of the Bible as God's word can never get rid of a lurking inner uncertainty, since every interpreter explains the Bible differently. Hence its authority is always in question; and it is no accident, though it is at the same time no proof of malevolent unbelief, that the absolute authority of the Bible has been questioned more and more by Protestant theologians ever since the Age of Enlightenment.

The attempt to invest the Bible with absolute authority in all religious matters, in the place of an hierarchical Church joined to the tremendous world of symbols, was a necessity of circumstance; but it was an inadequate attempt. If you must have a visible and tangible authority outside your own person, in the world at large, then the Catholic Church offers what is necessary in a form that can hardly be surpassed. Catholicism, it is true, also recognizes the Bible as an authority, but takes good care to interpret this authority as being grounded in another, and one which leaves no room for any uncertainties. In the papacy it has a living tribunal which—at the cost of submissive obedience—takes away all personal responsibility from the individual and guarantees him skilled and judicious guidance in all the vital questions. People who can find peace and certainty only in a church and only in an authority outside themselves will probably best attain it in the Catholic Church.

Parallel with this collapse of authority there is the disintegration of all the symbols taken over by Protestantism. The sacraments are all being taken more and more semiotically. The office of minister is losing all trace of the priestliness it once had. The ceremonial robes are vanishing. Belief in devils and witches is a thing of the past. Whatever we once—thanks to the conservatism of the Reformers—had in common with Catholicism is being given up. Neo-Protestantism, as the Protestantism of the post-Enlightenment period has been called ever since Ernst Troeltsch, has consistently liquidated the last vestiges of the Catholic outlook. The process went forward step by step and with a logic of its own. Neo-Protestantism has enabled the psychological attitude which led to the Reformation to emerge in full force. Today many people have gone so far that they have taken back their unconscious projections almost completely.[42]

This has had various results. First of all, it is now possible for modern man to have a much more frank, unbiased, and altogether clearer view of reality. Nature and history become accessible to him to a degree that did not exist before. So long as the individual projects his unconscious into the world at large, he is incapable of building up any scientific knowledge of his environment. Everything he does, when he tries to grasp the world as he then sees it, is no more than projected—unconscious—psychology. An example of this is alchemy. But the moment he ceases to project his unconscious, the picture he has of the world is emptied of its psychic contents, and he can then recognize the world for what it is, in so far as this is possible for the human mind at all. He is able to keep the images coming from his own psyche, and from the objects around him, strictly apart. He can tell the difference between phenomenon and the thing-in-itself. Modern science became possible only when the appearances of nature ceased to be vehicles for various kinds of psychic contents. But, because of this

[42] PR, p. 149.

withdrawal of psychic projections, the world becomes disenchanted. All the same, a world disenchanted of spirits and demons can be known much more objectively than when unconscious contents are always standing between man and reality.

The same is true of the "humane" sciences. The science of history, for instance, emerges only when historical events cease to be tangled up in mythology and can be examined soberly, without the play of unconscious elements. For Protestant theology, in particular, it was only with the cessation of the projection of unconscious contents on to the figure of Jesus that scholars could recognize and understand the historical Jesus. So long as Jesus is essentially a faith-symbol he cannot be seen historically. Those for whom Christ is a living religious symbol in the sense intended by Jung's psychology have no interest in any historical knowledge of Jesus of Nazareth; and even if they tried to know him they could not, because the symbolic value of the Christ-image would interpose itself between them and the Jesus of history. Only when the projection of religious contents on to the Jesus-figure has ceased can one set about historical research with any prospect of success. Protestantism has certainly made good use of the opportunities offered. During the nineteenth century Protestant theology achieved mighty feats of research in the field of Church history and dogma, in the historico-critical approach to the Old and New Testaments, in the life of Jesus, and in the history of religions. There is a whole series of works by Protestant theologians which are classics of scientific historiography. One has only to think of Harnack's *History of Dogma* or Albert Schweitzer's *Quest of the Historical Jesus*. Theology's achievements in this respect, like scientific research itself, are in the last resort the outcome of the Protestant spirit which ousted that of the Middle Ages. Modern science in all its more humane forms, historical research in its manifold departments, the scientific theology of neo-Protestantism which not only collates the opinions of our forefathers but ventures to put fundamental questions and also to answer them, and finally modern psychology, all emerged in connexion with that attitude of mind which first found expression in the Reformation. These are incomparable achievements indeed.

But Jung draws attention, equally clearly and discriminatingly, to the reverse side of this transformation. The spiritual and psychological crisis may have given rise to a matchless knowledge of the world, but a considerable price had to be paid. The symbols of earlier ages are now symbols no longer; they have ceased to work. Consequently, the unconscious cannot be projected on to them and exteriorized. But at the same time Protestantism forfeits the salvation that is given to those who know living symbols. The barriers that the Catholic Church erected against the unconscious, and in the shelter of which the true Catholic was immune to the perils of the soul, are down; hence the Protestant is delivered up to these psychic powers in a way that does not make life at all easy for him.[43] He has to reckon with the fact that the psychic elements which the Catholic, like the primitive man, reads into his surroundings are really there in his own soul.

With the abandonment of belief in the devil, the projection of the devil may be at an end, but the autonomous complex which man had read into the devilish image is still there—and, moreover, as a fact of inner experience. Previously, one could ascribe temptation

43 Ibid., p. 36; EJ 1934, p. 203.

to diabolical promptings and could try to exorcize it by means of magic and conjurations, but now the same old temptations are experienced as perils of the soul, and simples are not so easily had. On the contrary, modern man, Protestants and their pastors included, is powerless against them. It is not just a matter of the individual: the universal catastrophes of wars and revolutions all come, in Jung's view, from the breaking loose of unconscious forces. "If it [Protestantism] keeps on disintegrating as a Church, it must have the effect of stripping man of all his safeguards and means of defence, which shield him from the immediate experience of the forces waiting for liberation in the unconscious. Look at the incredible savagery of our so-called civilized world: it all comes from human beings and the spiritual condition they are in! Look at the diabolical means of destruction! They are invented by completely innocuous gentlemen—by reasonable, respectable citizens who are everything we could wish. And when the whole thing blows up and an indescribable hell of destruction is let loose, nobody seems to be responsible. It just happens, and yet it is all man-made. But since everybody is blindly convinced that he is nothing *more* than his own extremely unassuming and insignificant conscious mind, which performs its duties decently and earns him a moderate living, not a soul realizes that this whole rationally organized conglomeration we call the 'state' or 'nation' is driven on by what appears to be an impersonal, invisible, but terrible power which nothing and nobody can check. This frightful power is generally explained as fear of the neighbouring nation, which is supposed to be possessed by some malevolent fiend. Since nobody is capable of recognizing just where and how strongly he himself is possessed and unconscious, we all project our own state of mind on to our neighbours; and so it becomes a sacred duty to possess the biggest guns and the most poisonous gas. The worst of it is that we are all quite right. All our neighbours are in the grip of some uncontrolled an uncontrollable fear, just like ourselves."[44]

The individual's neuroses likewise prove that there are many persons who are incapable of establishing the kind of relationship with their unconscious which would enable them to live without spiritual dangers. Individuals as well as societies are riddled with fears—fear of the unconscious forces. Fear arises when an essential part of the psyche cannot be assimilated to the conscious mind, and when the individual is confronted with some inner discord that he cannot at the moment overcome. *Consequently, Protestantism is a great spiritual adventure.* It demolishes the symbols and projections which shield men from the unconscious. It thus takes a formidable risk, for at this juncture the "night-world of the soul" makes itself irresistibly felt. The Catholic can seek refuge from the sinister side of spiritual experience in Mother Church, but the Protestant, for whom the Church is psychologically a mother no longer, is defenceless.[45] We must add with all emphasis that this is an act of fate. Jung says: "This whole development is fate. I would lay the blame neither on Protestantism nor on the Renaissance. One thing, however, is certain: modern man, Protestant or not, has largely lost the protection of the ecclesiastical walls put up and fortified so carefully since Roman days, and because of this loss has come a little closer to the zone of the world-destroying and world-creating fire. Life has become faster and more intense. Our world rocks, shot through with uneasiness and fear."[46]

[44] *PR*, p. 88 f.　　　[45] *BZIU*, p. 145.　　　[46] *PR*, p. 88.

The condition of the Protestant can best be described as one of *spiritual poverty*.[47] Modern man stands alone, having reached a very high degree of consciousness,[48] but because of his lack of religion he is faced with religious problems. If the conscious mind cannot succeed in accommodating itself to a living religion or confession, then the religious question will be broached from the unconscious. The only thing is that this makes it more difficult. Even Protestant theologians are fairly helpless when faced with such a situation,[49] and Jung finds it highly remarkable, if also characteristic, that some of them are turning in their bewilderment to Freudian psychoanalysis.[50] Ultimately, even theologians cannot close their eyes to the fact that the so-called Christianity of today has largely become ineffectual.[51] Spitteler has caricatured traditional Christianity in his *Lämmchen* (Little Lamb)—not without reason.[52] Kierkegaard too testifies to the religious impoverishment of the present.[53] Jung sees the failure of contemporary Christianity in its manifest lack of individual culture. We can create a collective culture, but not a culture of individuals; and this gives rise to the disunity from which modern man is clearly suffering.[54] The Christian principle of love has led in practice to a completely extraverted attitude, which now looks for salvation—for when individual culture is lacking, the individual has the feeling that he is being sacrificed (Schiller). The last days of the Roman Empire were just the opposite: then there was individual culture but no collective culture. A

[47] *EJ 1934*, p. 192.
[48] *SPG*, p. 401.
[49] *Die Beziehungen der Psychotherapie zur Seelsorge*, p. 10.
[50] *WS*, p. 125.
[51] *Ibid.*, p. 63.
[52] *PT*, p. 263.
[53] *EJ 1934*, p. 185.
[54] *PT*, p. 103.

discrepancy made itself felt there too—hence the saving effect of Christianity.

In view of this interpretation, Jung cannot regard modern man and particularly the modern Protestant as "unreligious" in the ordinary sense. His voice has no part in the wail that is raised on all sides about the irreligiousness of modern man. On the contrary, he is firmly convinced that, consciously or unconsciously, the religious question is extremely acute and pressing for the Protestant of today. He finds that in patients of over thirty-five years of age religious problems are, without exception, vital and that ultimately it is these problems which induce people to see a psychotherapist. The Protestant goes because, the projection having ceased, the psychic elements contained in it are lost to him.[55] The quest may at first disguise itself in non-religious garb, but when one reaches the core of the questions which weigh on the minds of those in the second half of life, one invariably comes upon religious themes. Jung also states that it was his patients who compelled him to busy himself with the history of dogma and religion, and to acquire the knowledge he now has of religious symbolism. In the modern Protestant, therefore, Jung sees a man for whom traditional religion and the Christian creed have become questionable or, indeed, inoperative, but who for that very reason is forced to come to terms with the religious problem in some personal way.

Hence it is only very seldom that the Protestant turns atheist. If he leaves the Church he joins a sect; but the Catholic is more likely to become an atheist.[56] In the last resort the Protestant of today, even when he is on the

[55] *SPG*, p. 172.   [56] *PR*, p. 38.

point of quitting the Church or has actually done so, is only seeking religious experience. He is not seeking authority, because the psychological conditions for belief in authority are lacking. Jung says that it is characteristic of modern man that an "imitation of Christ" is no longer possible for him,[57] because he does not want an imitation of the past but self-experience and self-conviction. That is why a modern religious movement like anthroposophy styles itself not a "church" but a "humane science," thus hoping to stress the experiential side of it.

What, then, in Jung's view lies closest to modern man is the sort of procedure practised by the Gnostics—that sect which emerged in the early days of Christianity and combined Christianity with the spirit of antiquity. The Gnostics did not want to appropriate the symbols, ideas, and philosophy of the early Christians merely by recognizing their value; what they wanted was "gnosis" (knowledge) of them—that is, they wanted to *experience* their meaning and to make it conscious. From gnosticism onwards this tendency continued to make itself felt again and again in various esoteric or semi-esoteric sects, and the gnostic attitude to Christian dogma and symbolism is also apparent in the alchemists. Many moderns feel exactly the same way about the Christian tradition: they want not only to believe the truth of the symbols and venerate them, they also want to experience them and convince themselves of their truth. In this there is a struggle to approach closer to the unconscious, for whoever tries to become conscious of the actual content of the religious symbol is making a portion of the unconscious conscious at the same time. In this way he acquires living experience, and possibly religious experi-

[57] *Die Beziehungen der Psychotherapie zur Seelsorge*, p. 20.

ence too in a sense other than that intended by orthodox dogma—for the unconscious does not allow anybody to say in advance what it shall produce. Hence the way of gnosis is not without its dangers, a fact known not only to psychology but proved by practical experience in all gnostic communities.

As we have hinted, a man may take the "gnostic" way when he is engrossed in some psychic problem. This is still the case in our own times, and according to Jung the spiritual problem of modern man is the problem of evil.[58] The Catholic, standing firm in his Church, can solve the problem of evil quite easily; he projects it into Satan and can free himself of guilt by confessing. The Protestant, however, cannot project evil; consequently, he experiences it in himself and cannot get rid of it in the confessional. He has to tackle it personally. Hence he may in certain circumstances feel evil and ugliness as the antichrist. He experiences the problem of opposites in his own self. Theology has always been concerned with this problem, e.g. in the theodicy theory, which was born of man's contradictory experience of himself and the world. But there is no final solution of it in modern theology, and accordingly an eloquent silence reigns far and wide over the theodicy problem. For these reasons theology is not in a position to help when the individual experiences evil as a reality in the world or even in himself. The symbols no longer work, and theology has no remedy. The situation of the "Protestant person" is therefore this: he feels a deep discord—a sharp antithesis and a correspondingly deep need of salvation—but can find no way out of his dilemma. Hence that anxiety which plays so prominent a part in many forms of present-day Christianity and their theologies.

[58] *SPG*, p. 414.

There has, however, been no lack of attempts to find a way out. For the present situation and the anxiety associated with it have begun to cause discomfort to many Protestants, theologians and non-theologians alike. One solution is the demand for a belief in the traditional symbols and dogmas, even if the "believer" experiences no immediate saving effect. The symbols and dogmas had this effect once—that is historically correct; therefore, it is argued, perhaps it can be induced once more. Belief of this kind is interpreted as submission to "saving truth," and the price required is the *sacrificium intellectus*. In canonical Protestantism this procedure leads to the so-called "repristination" theology, which holds fast to the store of dogmas and symbols taken over by the Reformers from Catholicism and tries by hook or by crook to persuade men that they will feel saved if only they acknowledge the truth of these. Symptomatic, too, is the recurrent appeal to fear—a favourite device of ecclesiastical propaganda in this revival of Protestant orthodoxy (and with certain advocates of Catholicism, too).

Jung thinks nothing of such a belief, for, according to it, one must believe not only in the symbols and dogmas themselves but also in their saving effect.[59] This, however, is not the way the living symbol works, which, if it is indeed a living thing, saves more by virtue of its livingness than by any belief in it. The living symbol brings about a union of opposite tensions; this is an empirically recognizable result and never merely an object of "belief." When submission to the symbols and dogmas of faith is demanded, the result is only religiosity; for the submission can be made for all sorts of reasons, none of which accords with the psychic value of

[59] *WSL*, p. 277.

the symbols and dogmas in question. What is experienced in this kind of "salvation" may have all the appearance of genuine religious salvation, but is of slight effect and in time proves insignificant. Generally speaking, it is a matter of psychic processes which other people can equally well experience or induce outside religion; which can therefore never be called specifically religious and, for anybody acquainted with genuine religious experience, are obviously in a different class. Hence faith in this sense has nothing in common with real religion and is an experiment that holds out no prospect of success, because it is psychologically impossible to succeed.

The Victorian Age, not only in England but on the Continent as well, was loud in professing this kind of faith; it was the last great effort to maintain the religious ideas and ideals of the Middle Ages.[60] It ended in a completely bogus and spiritually vapid sort of sanctimoniousness, the reasons for which are psychologically all too obvious. One cannot, with the best will in the world and the strongest measures of coercion, force psychological facts to go backwards. Otherwise, the Inquisition would have been able to check this whole trend five hundred years ago. Psychologically, again, this return to the symbols of the past is a typical regression. When people try to put old ecclesiastical wine into new ecclesiastical bottles it is a sure sign of religious crisis. They are confronted with a situation that is extremely difficult to master, and they attempt to solve the problems of the present with the psychic instruments of an earlier age.[61] But the difficulties of the present can only be mastered by devising the measures that are appropriate to them. No more than the individual can solve the

[60] *WS*, p. 120.   [61] *PT*, p. 266.

problems of old age by recapturing the attitude of his youth, can the religious crisis of today be solved by a return to the earlier remedies. The present must be experienced for what it is, and any repetition of an old attitude is mere escapism.

The other way out is to borrow such help as we need from the non-Christian religions. If the way we have just described is an evasion in time, this is an evasion in space. It is, as we know, widely practised today. People make the discovery that the Oriental religions contain living symbols which equip the Oriental with the means of salvation. Alien peoples find in their religion what they need, and maybe we can too. Hence many try to adopt these symbols in the hope of being saved. This *Drang nach Osten* in quest of religious help started with Schopenhauer, and it is still going strong. Jung rejects this solution. For we are, after all, men of the West, and as soon as we really try to understand the men of the East we notice the abysmal difference between us. The Oriental is as incomprehensible to us as we are to him.[62] The difference can be defined in brief thus: The Oriental has a real spiritual culture, whereas we are the barbarians of the soul. Instead, we have attained a degree of consciousness and knowledge of the world unknown to the Oriental. Jung sees no reason for us to give up this advantage. On the contrary, the religious symbols of the East, coming as they do from a living spiritual culture, are bound to remain incomprehensible in the end and ineffective as far as *our* souls are concerned. Jung has often been suspected of recommending Oriental practices whereby the individual might effect his own salvation, and of himself taking part in this flight to the East. His keen interest in Oriental religions has inevitably led to such a

[62] Jung-Suzuki: *Die grosse Befreiung*, p. 9.

verdict. But if he is a student of Oriental religions, it is only because he finds certain psychic processes clearly described there—processes which also exist in the West but which the Oriental, thanks to his being better acquainted with what is going on inside him, can express more vividly.

How Jung views the use of Oriental religions by Westerners and what solution he regards as the right one for the "Protestant person" of today is shown by the following passage: "I am convinced that it is not for nothing that the Protestant person has, as it were, been stripped naked by his development. This development has an inner logic of its own. All the things that meant nothing to him in his thoughts have been stripped away. If he should now go and wrap his nakedness in the gorgeous trappings of the Orient, as the theosophists do, he would be playing his own history false. One does not conduct oneself as a beggar only to pose afterwards as an Indian potentate. Nor is there any need to go as far as the theosophists. There are more modest ways of compensating for the loss of Christian symbolism. Nevertheless, it is a substitute, a mere exchange of symbols, and it remains just as dark as before precisely *what* primordial experiences are being expressed through the symbols.

"It seems to me that it would be far better stoutly to avow our spiritual poverty, our symbol-lessness, instead of feigning a legacy to which we are not the legitimate heirs at all. We are the rightful heirs of Christian symbolism, but somehow we have squandered this heritage. We have let the house our fathers built fall into decay, and now we try to break into palaces that our fathers never knew. Why do we not say instead: 'We are poor,' and be serious for once with that famous trust in God we are always prating of. But if ever it comes to the point, we stay God's arm and want to manage by ourselves, not only *as if* we were afraid but because we are, in actual fact, devilishly afraid things would then go wrong. . . . This fear is anything but unjustified, for where God is closest the danger is greatest. It is dangerous to avow spiritual poverty, for the poor man has desires, and whoever has desires calls down some fatality on himself. A Swiss proverb puts it drastically like this: 'Behind every rich man there is a devil, and behind a poor man two!' Just as in Christianity the vow of worldly poverty turned the mind away from the riches of this earth, so spiritual poverty seeks to renounce the false riches of the spirit in order to withdraw not only from the pathetic remnants—which call themselves the Protestant Church—of a great past, but also from all the allurements of the odorous East; in order, finally, to commune with our own selves, where, in the cold light of consciousness, the blank barrenness of the world reaches to the very stars." [63] And he goes on: "Whoever has elected for the state of spiritual poverty, which is the true heritage of a Protestantism carried to its logical conclusion, goes the way of the soul that leads to the water. This water is no figure of speech, but a living symbol created by the soul itself." [64] It is the way into the unconscious.

So that in this psychological crisis Jung sees no possibility of retreat or evasion. For him it is only a way of carrying the present spiritual situation to its end: the way into the soul, the way to self-experience. Because the Protestant is stripped bare of traditional symbols it is possible for him to have this experience. And only from primordial experience can true faith come again.[65]

[63] *EJ 1934*, p. 192.   [64] *Ibid.*, p. 195.   [65] *SPG*, p. 85.

188

Faith is a gift (*charisma*) which the primordial religious experience grants to man. Jung points to the apostle Paul by way of proof that we can overcome our spiritual suffering and heal our inner disunity only through experience of the self. Paul became a Christian only because he had first actualized and experienced his loathing of Christians.[66] Had he not given vent to this hatred he would never have become a Christian. Theoretical considerations are of no help in a situation like this, only experience serves. The fact that the symbolism of the Church no longer protects the Protestant from his own unconscious is his peculiar danger, but it is also his great and unique opportunity.[67] The dissolution of symbols exposes him to the risk of losing all spiritual orientation and certainty, but at the same time he may gain the primordial religious experience—if he makes direct contact with the unconscious.

"The Protestant is left to God alone. For him there is no confession, no absolution, no possibility of an expiatory *opus divinum* of any kind. He has to digest his sins by himself; and, because the absence of a suitable ritual has put it beyond his reach, he is none too sure of God's grace. Hence the present alertness of the Protestant conscience—and this bad conscience has all the unpleasant characteristics of a lingering illness which makes people chronically uncomfortable. But because of this the Protestant has a unique chance to realize his sin to a degree that is beyond the reach of the Catholic mentality, since confession and absolution are always at hand to ease excess of tension. The Protestant, however, is left to his tensions, which can go on sharpening his conscience. Conscience, and in particular a bad conscience,

---

[66] *Die Beziehungen der Psychotherapie zur Seelsorge*, p. 9.
[67] *PR*, p. 89 f.

can be a gift of heaven, a veritable grace if used in the interests of the higher self-criticism. And self-criticism, in the sense of an introspective, discriminating activity, is essential in every effort to understand one's own psychology. When we have done something that seems inexplicable, and we ask ourselves what could have induced us to do it, we need the sting of a bad conscience and the powers of discrimination that go with it, in order to discover the real motives of our behaviour. Only thus do we become capable of seeing what motives dominate our actions. A bad conscience spurs us on to discover things that before were unconscious, and in this way we can cross the threshold of the unconscious and take cognizance of those impersonal forces which make us the unconscious instrument of the mass-murderer in man. If a Protestant survives the complete loss of his Church and still remains a Protestant - that is, a person who is defenceless against God and no longer protected by walls or communities—then he has a unique spiritual opportunity for immediate religious experience." [68]

Protestant man's "opportunity," then, is the possibility he has of experiencing what Jung calls "individuation." We would refer to what was said above on this head. The resultant widening of personality is a tremendous gain for the individual; and the experience may well crystallize out into a new God-image, into an access of religious feeling through which new and surprising elements may be assimilated. In the dream-series that Jung has used in various publications [69] one gets some inkling of the process, but also of what it costs. It is not for nothing that Jung emphasizes that it needs "all kinds of courage"—not to speak of *religio*, i.e. a careful consider-

[68] *Ibid.*, pp. 89 ff.
[69] *EJ 1935; Psychology and Religion; Psychology and Alchemy*, etc.

ation of supra-personal forces—to follow the road to its end. It requires considerable courage to accept oneself just as one is, to face up to oneself. Also, the approach to the unconscious may give rise to panic terror. It is no accident that when his personal experience of God threatened to become too dangerous Angelus Silesius almost fell over himself to get into the Catholic Church in order to escape the unconscious powers.

Jung is not to be taken as recommending this path to everybody. Only a very superficial knowledge of his psychology could lead to such a conclusion. It is definitely not a matter of experiments that can be undertaken at will, or from boredom, or for amusement. In that case, either one would completely miss the point, perhaps to one's own advantage, or one would be toying with one's psychic equilibrium very frivolously indeed. Where another solution exists, Jung would always recommend it. On the other hand, there are certain people to whom he could advise only the way of self-experience. There are people today who are spiritually fragmented and who have a distinct feeling that all is not well. They sense that they are not satisfying the demands of life, and their life does not satisfy them either. They are aware of perpetual discord and are appalled at the meaninglessness of their existence. They suffer from a fear that is grounded in their psychic constellation. They need a rebirth of soul, and this is to be attained only through the sort of psychic wholeness we described earlier. That this should be intended for them is their fate, and no light one at that; but there is no escape from fate save by the acceptance of it. Jung sees it as an absolute necessity for them to satisfy this demand for psychic wholeness, and as a pastor of souls, in the widest sense of the word, he can only direct his efforts to shepherding them along this path. In his lecture "Psychotherapy and the Cure of Souls", he uses a formula that sounds very simple: man must accept himself. The point for the Protestant Christian is that he must live his own life and remain true to himself as Christ lived his own life and remained true to himself.

There are many people today whom orthodox religious symbolism can no longer help because there has been a change in the collective psyche. A portion of it, hitherto repressed by Christianity, is stirring and asserting itself. This portion Jung calls the "Dionysian element." At the same time Jung thinks that, even with Nietzsche and afterwards, the term "Dionysus" was only such as would naturally occur to the classical philologist, but that what was really in question was Wotan, the god of storm.[70] The mysteries of Dionysus gave men a re-connexion (religion) with nature, and of this nature man must now become conscious: as the nature innate in his own soul.[71]

Jung has no intention of creating a new religion for Protestant man, being fully persuaded that Christianity is the specific religion of the West. That does not necessarily mean Christianity in its traditional form. In his *Psychology and Alchemy*, Jung says that Christianity in general and Protestantism in particular must absorb more of the spirit of Meister Eckhart. For the projection of religious experience into the world at large, away from man, is injurious both to man and to religion. It creates a vacuum in the soul, and the result is a lull in spiritual development. The Reformation was a break in the sovereignty of the Catholic Church. But at the same time it was only a transition stage. To continue the Reformation, however, it is not enough to go on reforming and modifying the Church to which it gave birth. For Jung the Reformed

[70] *EJ 1935*, pp. 69, 74; *Neue Schweizer Rundschau 1936*, No. 11.
[71] *PR*, pp. 50, 52.

Church, viewed historically, is significant only in that it has taught us Christians that a religious mode of life is possible not merely within the setting of an all-powerful Church, built in wisdom and cunningly planned in all its details, but as personal experience. Our task now, says Jung, is to let this development go forward, stripping off the last vestiges of ecclesiasticism that cling to the Protestant Church—which means that the individual must himself be the bearer of further changes and new religious experiences. A new religious pattern of life must replace the one broken down by the Reformation. This new pattern of religious experience will be individual. It will, in Jung's view, be Christian but not ecclesiastical. Because the Protestant feels the problems thrown up by the disintegration of the old religious symbols and the Church as *personal* problems, *personal* troubles and difficulties, as a disharmony and inner conflict felt in his own person, there can only be personal solution and salvation, and this demands a *personal* stake. Jung sees it as one of the essential tasks of his psychotherapy to make the individual aware of this need for inward reconstruction, and to help him fulfil this need. He tries to do that in the one place where the individual has immediate experience: in the soul. So that ultimately his aim is to put us, through the soul, directly in touch with the powers which create and transform life itself.

When Jung stresses the fact that he only came to religious problems through his patients, we can lay it down as a corollary that it is essentially *because of* the religious development of Western man that we have a psychology and a psychotherapy today. Because many people could not find a psychic foothold, as it were, in the traditional Christian symbolism, nor express themselves in those terms, they were driven to the realization of certain psychic factors. These forced themselves on their consciousness, and it is simply a consequence of this inner development that we now have a scientific psychology of the unconscious. Strange as it may seem at first, the evolution of Christianity itself is for Jung the prime cause of that urge to self-knowledge, the scientific form of which is psychology. We can therefore understand why it is that Jung always sends patients back to the Catholic Church and the confessional if at all possible. But we can also understand why this cannot invariably be so, and why there are people who need a pastor with no confessional ties to help them along the road to self-knowledge. And it is clear, too, why a great many Protestants should go to a pastor with a psychological rather than a theological training in their troubles. In his lecture to the Alsatian Society of Ministers Jung made known the results of an interesting inquiry into this question.[72]

If psychology is born of the urge to self-knowledge and of the distressed condition of religion today, something else becomes understandable—namely, why Jung, the Protestant pastor's son, turned psychologist. He tells the story himself: "I still remember well my confirmation and the preliminary instruction I received at my father's hands. The catechism bored me unspeakably. One day I was turning over the pages of my little book, in the hope of finding something interesting, when my eye fell on the paragraphs about the Trinity. This interested me at once, and I looked forward with impatience for the lessons to get to that section. But when the longed-for day came my father said, 'We'll skip this bit; I can't make head or tail of it myself.' With that my last hopes were dashed."[73] Hence it would seem to be no accident if the

[72] *Die Beziehungen der Psychotherapie zur Seelsorge.*
[73] *EJ* 1934, p. 193.

pastor's son decided against a course of theological study without any qualms or inner struggles and became a doctor and psychiatrist, but made up for it later, as a psychologist, by writing whole volumes steeped in theological lore on such questions as whether the Trinity or the Quaternity of God best corresponds to the structure of the soul!

Of course, there is more to it than that—above all, Jung's unqualified zest for life, which is part of his unbounded desire to help people in their spiritual distresses. He sees that the spiritual distress of today is world-wide. For it is not only those who consult the doctor or psychotherapist on account of some definite spiritual problem that need help; it is also the man who shares the immense bewilderment of the present age, and of these there are very many. To these people, whose life has lost its meaning perhaps without their noticing it, but who can no longer help themselves when faced with the crucial questions, Jung would point a way. Such a way to spiritual healing and health Jung sees in religion, the very field of human life where our modern aimlessness is so acutely felt that many people turn away from it, thinking that nothing of any value is to be found there. But Jung, in his investigation of the unconscious, soon hit on the psychic elements that led him straight to religion. Thus it is that he recognizes more and more clearly the importance for the soul of a living religion, and that is why he draws religion more and more into the field of his activities as a healer in the widest sense of the word. Behind Jung's affirmative attitude to religion there stands his great, helpful affirmation of life, which, quite apart from his encyclopaedic scientific knowledge, is one of the most impressive things about him.

JUNG'S SIGNIFICANCE IN THE RELIGIOUS SITUATION OF TODAY

IN CONCLUSION, let us make an attempt to assess Jung's significance in the religious situation of today, particularly from the Protestant standpoint. An attempt it must remain, and nothing more, if only for the reason that it is very difficult if not impossible to judge the unfinished work of a living writer. Further, the author lacks competence to pass any valid judgement on Jung's especial province: psychology. Thus, what we now present is a number of suggestions and problems which, in the author's eyes, seem to emerge from Jungian psychology, with a view to a more explicit formulation of certain points that were all the time implied in the foregoing exposition.

The reader who has borne in mind Jung's utterances on the subject of religion will probably object that they are teeming with contradictions. Now one thing is said, now another; and as soon as one thinks that one has at last found a definitive statement to hold on to, a few pages further on one discovers the exact opposite. If the reader, more especially the theologically trained reader, objects that this exposition is riddled with contradictions, nothing could please the author more, since he will then see that he has succeeded in giving a more or less faithful account of Jung's religious psychology. For the contradictions do not derive from the author, but from Jung himself. It is Jung who is full of praise for a rigidly dogmatic and hierarchical Church and who in the same book counsels those who want personal experience of religion to quit the Church. It is Jung who praises the wisdom and beauty of ecclesiastical dogma and immediately after, to prove his thesis, cites heretics and heresiarchs whom the Fathers of the Church—the very men who created the dogma—condemned as the Devil's brood. It is Jung who sends people back into the Catholic Church so that the confessional shall protect them from the dangers of introspection and then extols Meister Eckhart, who rescued God, heaven, and hell from projection into the world at large and lodged them in his own soul, thereby stimulating the intensive study of the self and the world within. It is Jung who warns against laying so much as a finger on dogma and whose psychology consistently attacks all submission to orthodoxy in the sense of a *sacrificium intellectus*. Indeed, it can truly be said that Jung's whole psychology is one long protest against the acceptance of Christian dogma in this way, which, though supported by all strict ecclesiastics of whatever confession, always demands the sacrifice of a part of the human soul together with that of the intellect and is thus diametrically opposed to Jung's ultimate aims. One could multiply these contradictions *ad libitum;* they will certainly not have escaped the attentive reader. Everybody who plunges into Jungian psychology will come up against them and must therefore reckon with them beforehand.

For many people, theologians in particular and perhaps the philosophically-minded as well, such contradictions are not easy to put up with. We hear it said that Jung may be a good enough doctor but that he is certainly no scientific thinker. In fact, there are to my knowledge persons who accuse Jung of dishonesty on this account and say that he acts on the principle of the bad judge who pronounced all the litigants, one after another, right in the same affair, not excluding the man who drew his attention to what he was doing. We even hear Jung accused of playing to the gallery, currying favour, etc., so as to keep in the good graces of everybody.

Now, it is right to fix on his contradictions: they *do* exist. But to attribute them to defects in Jung's character or to accuse him of being unscientific is quite another thing. Nor can it be justified in view of the real state of affairs in the sphere of religion. There are in fact numerous religions. All sorts of things occur on the plane of religious life, and it cannot be doubted that they are all very different. And is not the individual, too, anything but logical as regards religion, from the philosophical point of view? A man may believe in science on week-days, and on Sunday that Jesus rose bodily from the dead, that he was born of a virgin, and that the world was created in seven days, though a credo of this sort could hardly be squared with his scientific convictions. And another thing: theologians ordinarily have the peculiarity of regarding what they say as the absolute truth at that moment and of doubting the genuine Christianity of all those who do not share their views one hundred per cent. Two, three years later they take back a good part of it and replace it by other asseverations for which they make exactly the same claims. One has only to think of the vehemence with which the convert inveighs against his former attitude. Since this is so, there is a regular spate of theological books, articles, and talks whose main object is to demonstrate the untruth of all other points of view and to laud only those championed by the author. The East, as is well known, has a very different procedure. There, it is quite natural for people to belong to different religious communities between the official doctrines of which there are differences of the same magnitude as those existing between the Christian confessions. The Indian or Japanese goes beyond these differences, picking out the good he can find in the various creeds and taking what he needs from each. Never yet has any European, theologian or otherwise, put forward any plausible reason why this Oriental attitude to the fact that there are many kinds of religious faith should be worse, in an absolute sense, than the European one, which leads to everlasting struggles and squabbles. At all events, noteworthy reasons could easily be advanced for the other procedure.

On the surface Jung's attitude to religion is more in keeping with the Eastern than the Western view. But the reasons for this are certainly not those of the Oriental. Jung is a psychologist and follows the dictates of the psyche. Therefore he starts from the assumption, right in itself, that every religious attitude and every faith, whatever it be, must have its psychological reasons. The psychologist, and particularly the psychotherapist, must first accept man as he is. He cannot set up as a judge, only as a helper; and to help he must first understand. But understanding implies recognizing and approving a man in his peculiarities. Jung never fails to give us a reason as to why he approves or recommends a particular course of action. He says quite clearly that he would not send every patient who was a Catholic back to the Catholic Church, and that he would not recommend personal religious experience to everybody without exception. It depends on the individual and not on systems of logic whether Jung approaches the religious question and offers the patient guidance in this respect. The primary thing for him is the individual soul; and the theologian, of all people, should know, if he has any serious appreciation of the various religions with which his theological studies should have acquainted him, just how irrational and ambiguous an entity the soul is. It is for this reason that the religions vary so much in their form and content. There is no point in accusing Jung of being illogical and contradictory, for the good reason that this lies in the diversity of religion itself. And all dogma which tries to get rid of this diversity only ends by adding yet another dogmatism to it. If one cannot accept Jung's views for oneself, at least one can admit that Jung, as a psychologist, has the right to let himself be influenced by the great number of religions and their inner differences, and to try to be fair to them all.

All Jung's ideas about religion either are very novel or fit in with those of people who have been branded as heretics and cranks by the orthodox Church. It is scarcely possible, therefore, for everybody to agree with him. However that may be, one thing above all should be stressed: Jung's ideas are not the result of mere theory or of historical research—they have been wrested from the hard facts of his psychotherapeutic practice. Jung is not one of those psychologists who has a chair in psychology somewhere and gleans his knowledge—with more or less discrimination—in odd nooks and crannies; he is, by profession, a medical pastor of souls, and, year in year out, hundreds of people come to him with their psychological difficulties, their troubles and worries, their thoughts and experiences. And not only that: he must, in one way or another, help them. Thus, he not only possesses a very deep insight into the spiritual life of modern man; he has also to look round for what can help these sufferers.

It is true that Jung's clientele today comes almost exclusively from a certain class, and one that is highly cultivated. But we all know that spiritual movements and ideas have always in the end filtered through to all the classes in the population. Some ideas are seized on more quickly than others, yet when a certain complex of experience is not merely the product of a lone, original thinker, when it has the power to seize on a whole group, perhaps only one particular stratum of society at first, in time it will penetrate everywhere. Such experiences are consequently not unimportant. And if people are at all interested in the vocation of minister or in religion, they will do well to acquaint themselves with Jung. For it is absolutely certain that, sooner or later, they will have to come to terms with him. It is not the facts alone that help to shape Jung's views, his interpretation of the facts also plays an important part; and Jung is a self-willed and altogether extraordinary thinker who is apt to construe certain things very differently from other scientists. But this is not to say in the least that we need not bother with his interpretation of the facts. On the contrary, just because he is a psychologist and psychotherapist who has to get to know his patients in the most personal way, he is to be listened to and reckoned with very seriously indeed. For it is a well-known fact that the doctor's profession requires him to devote his whole personality to the patient to the fullest possible degree. The patient may be guided and moulded by the person of the doctor, but the doctor in his turn is always shaped and changed in the process. Consequently, even if Jung's scientific views reflect his own personal idiosyncrasies, they must still be given the most serious attention.

Many of Jung's ideas are, as a matter of fact, highly individual. But many of his ideas about religion have their counterpart in theology. Jung interprets the Reformation, as we have said, as iconoclasm in the sense that Catholicism, through its symbols, projects the whole complex of religious experience into the world at large, and the Reformation took the projection back again, thus devaluing the symbols. In his book *Das protestantische Prinzip in Kirche und Welt* (The Protestant Principle in the Church and World), Theodor Siegfried, starting from totally different assumptions and using an altogether different approach, comes to the same conclusion. He says that Luther *interiorized* heaven and hell, and in this way felt religious experience much more profoundly in his own soul than had been the case until then. That is essentially the same as what Jung says, even though Jung speaks of a lifting of psychological projection and Siegfried of a spiritualization of Catholic dogma.

To many people, at least in regard to religion, it may be objectionable to be told that all immediate religious experience is a psychic process and that this alone is the basis of any real religion. Here, too, we can find a parallel in modern Protestant theology. Hermann Lüdemann says much the same thing in his *Dogmatik*, and works on this principle entirely. He also says that self-experience is of prime importance for religion. This is all the more interesting in that Lüdemann, as those in any way familiar with him must know, is poles apart from Jung both in his hypotheses and in his methods. The basic agreement, therefore, is all the more significant. In this respect Jung has a strong affinity with the views of Schleiermacher, particularly those which have found little or no recognition in the Protestant theology of the last century.

When Jung says that the fundamental problem of modern man who is a Christian, in the widest sense of the word, is the nature, the naturalistic element inherent in the unconscious and the assimilation of this to personality, he finds an echo in the words of a theologian, Kurt Leese. In his interesting book *Die Krisis und Wende des christlichen Geistes* (The Crisis of Christianity), Leese comes, on the basis of an historical analysis, to the conclusion that the great problem for present-day theology—and we can cheerfully say for contemporary Christianity as a whole—is nature. He writes: "Are the days of Christianity numbered? Can we speak not only of a decline of the West, but of its God as well? Is a new *Götterdämmerung* about to begin? Only one lamentably ignorant of all the upheavals that are taking place deep down in life could be so rash as to see any profanity in these questions. Christian theologians, triumphantly falling back on Luther, Calvin, and Kierkegaard, have been indoctrinating us with the 'crisis of man,' the 'crisis of history,' the 'crisis of civilization,' the 'crisis of philosophy,' the 'crisis of religion,' etc., etc. What have they *not* questioned for God's sake? There was, indeed, little that could not be questioned in times that seemed to lack any sure standards. But what if the spearhead of their attack were to turn against themselves, what if there were a fundamental crisis of Christian theology, which is so cock-sure of itself? What if its God, far from being too great and paradoxical, were to prove too small and unparadoxical? . . . The Absolute Spirit of the idealist philosopher and the Holy Spirit of the apostle Paul may be as different as earth and heaven. Only, we have revelled too long in the consciousness of their contrariety. Where they both meet is precisely in the fact that they are *spirit* and not nature. . . . 'Nature,' if we are not wholly mistaken, is the great conundrum common to both idealist philosophy and Christian theology, and it is becoming more and more urgent and troublesome." [1]

As will be apparent from these introductory words, Leese's approach is completely different from Jung's, but there is significant agreement between them as regards the problem of nature and the experience of God. Moreover,

[1] *Op. cit.*, p. 1.

the words that Leese uses as a motto to his book can also be found in Jung. They are: *Nemo contra Deum nisi Deus ipse* (Nobody is against God save God himself).

True, the Protestant theologians we have quoted do not belong to the common run, for which reason they are not recognized in ecclesiastical circles. All the same, they will have served to show that one can, starting from theological premises, reach conclusions which tally with Jung's, and this corroboration by psychological and theological inquiry lends them all the more weight.

Since we are on theological ground here, we shall give prominence to certain of Jung's views which are not, perhaps, of marked importance either for him or for the majority of his readers, but which may be recommended to Protestant theologians in particular. We are referring to the *positive attitude* Jung has to the development of Christianity and of Protestantism itself. It has become the fashion in Protestant theology nowadays—and likewise in many other fields of intellectual life—for people to demonstrate the novelty and originality of their ideas by attacking other thinkers—sometimes whole historical periods—with a view to devaluing them as much as possible. Such people think that they have staked their claim to public notice only if they have massacred their rivals. It is all right for political careerists to go in for such tactics, but it arouses more misgivings when certain persons within the pale of Protestant theology cannot, it seems, do enough to decry neo-Protestantism—that is to say, the whole development of Protestantism from about 1700 right up to the present—thinking, as they do, that it is only by restoring the theology of the Reformation that they can be saved from ruin. We find it refreshing to read Jung in this connexion. For his psychology gives one a new understanding of Catholicism. This is needful, since for a very long time the Catholic Church was the sole representative of Christianity, and our forefathers were all Catholics. But it also gives us a new understanding of the Reformation and, indeed, of the most recent developments of Protestantism. We realize that it is no accident, but, on the contrary, a most significant development, that the dogmas and sacraments were pulled down and scientific knowledge arose in their stead. We come to see the reasons for this, we see every stage of the journey with its advantages and disadvantages, we see the outcome of it, and also the price that had to be paid. Speaking purely theologically, therefore, Jungian psychology means an enrichment of our knowledge that cannot be too highly estimated.

The theologian, of course, will see Jung's significance in relation to the cure of souls. Jung's is a medical curacy, and the curate's business also lies with the care and cure of the individual soul, albeit from the point of view of his church and his own religious creed. We shall be divulging no secrets when we say that, in this matter of the cure of souls, the theologian and clergyman have reached a dead end. For either pastoral work is merely a continuation of the sermon, and can thus result only in collective pronouncements which hardly affect the individual at all, or the clergyman, if he feels any obligations to the individual, will suddenly discover that the means at his disposal are inadequate. The Catholic priest is much more favourably situated, since he always has the protection of the Church behind him, which is no longer the case with the Protestant clergyman. The latter, too, is bound to have a far stronger sort of *personal* relationship with the man who wants spiritual help, and he has to cope personally with his demands, which are often extremely difficult. But the clergyman will never meet these demands by dogmatism and a little natural insight into human character. We need not say over-much about this crisis in the pastoral work of the Protestant clergy; Dr. O. Pfister, himself a clergyman, has said what is to the point.

Complex psychology can give the clergyman a number of aids which will equip him more adequately for his office than has been the case hitherto. Even Freudian psychoanalysis has something to offer him—if he really does aspire to be a pastor of souls - despite the repellent outer garb it must have for every theologian. And in spite of all critical reservations, it is obvious that nobody can plough through Freud without reaping some benefit. This is also true of Jung, and to a far higher degree. We cannot expatiate on this question here, but we would refer the reader to Jung's lecture before the Alsatian Society of Ministers on "Psychotherapy and the Cure of Souls." One or two points from it can, however, be stressed at once.

Jung lays it down as a fact of primary importance (and in this he is in full agreement with Freudian psychoanalysis) that there can be no curing the souls of other people without first treating your own soul. Psychoanalysis requires every psychotherapist who wants to apply Freudian techniques to be psychoanalysed himself. Jung categorically adopts the same view. Whether every practising clergyman can or should go as far as this is a question apart. Perhaps it would be best not to expect every clergyman to apply psychiatry to people who have deep-seated difficulties, but to leave this either to the medical psychotherapist or to the clergyman with special training. Even if this were done, there is still something essential in this requirement of Jung's. Probably no clergyman can really serve or help others unless he satisfies certain psychological requirements. A reasonable degree of self-knowledge must be there, not merely in the sense that he examines himself for overt or covert sins, as is quite natural in one particular theology, but in the sense that he has some insight into the motives and purposes of his own actions, his own attitude. Certain psychological causes are at work in the choice of the clerical profession. It is simple enough, and it sounds very fine, to make vague references to the Holy Ghost, but mostly it is beside the point. The discovery of the real reasons is the prime task of this self-knowledge. What is more, the inner motives—I might almost say the "archetypes," which fix the clergyman's attitude to his profession—must also be clarified in the course of time. Often more depends on this than on the theological trends which Protestant clergymen make such a fuss about today. At any rate, the clergyman follows a certain ecclesiastical trend not for theological reasons alone, since there are always psychological motives at the back of his choice. If theologians do not know this, and do not want to know it, such an attitude does not militate against a psychological interpretation of their hidden motives; on the contrary, it demands it with all the more force. Jung's psychology and Jaspers's book *Die Psychologie der Weltanschauungen* are so informative in this respect that it is impossible to be deceived about the real state of affairs even by the most skilful and tortuous formulations of theology.

The same methods should be applied to the parish. A clergyman's parish generally has a pretty accurate picture of what a clergyman ought to be, and his success or failure often depends on whether he comes up to this picture.

The relations between clergyman and parish are largely unconscious, hence a psychological clarification, which would reveal the unconscious aims and motives, is all the more necessary. A psychological study of the clergyman and his parish could easily be written in terms of Jungian psychology, and this must be done one day. It would show us quite clearly where we stand and what the psychological background is. Nor would it be a slight or undesirable thing if the clergyman had some idea of what the persona is and what it means when a man—perhaps the clergyman himself—hankers after psychic wholeness. Many of the inhibitions and inner constraints which are today inseparable from the office of clergyman, and which torment great numbers of them almost to death or at least turn them into spiritual cripples, to their own hurt and that of the people entrusted to their care, would thus be removed.

Jungian psychology would also bring the clergyman up against a problem which, strictly speaking, is one of the most important questions in the whole field of pastoral work at present: should the spiritual director pay more attention to the individual or to the community? Catholicism, demanding as it does that the individual should submit to the teachings and rulings of the Church, has opted exclusively for the primacy of the community. Protestantism is not at all united on this question, perhaps not very clear about it. Protestant theologians sometimes go so far as deliberately to give the individual and his spiritual welfare a back place, or to neglect him completely. The Church, they say, has to proclaim God's word, but she does not have to take up the woes of the individual. God's word should cover everything that is salutary for the individual, and the theologian need not bother about anything else. One cannot rid oneself of the suspicion, however, that behind this attitude there lurks no real understanding but only vast confusion. People do not know what to do with the individual and how to answer his importunate demands. Be that as it may, the fact remains that even the most cursory glance at psychology shows that the individual soul is of supreme importance.

Jung, who advocates individuation in the case of certain people and wants to help everybody to find the religion he needs, expresses himself in no uncertain terms about the necessity for the individual approach. Since his psychology opens up the pastoral problem in its religious aspect, it is fitting to give the matter due consideration. At all events this question can no longer be ignored or fobbed off with dogmatic assertions. Obviously, no one form of religion can satisfy *everybody*. Moreover Jung says, from long years of psychotherapeutic experience, that there are people today who actually need personal experience of religion, and for whom, therefore, the doctrines of the Church or the community cannot possibly give what they most require. It is useless to object that such people are few and far between—the fact that they exist at all is significant. Jung advocates personal experience not for the sake of a pallid religiosity which combines elements drawn from all sorts of religions; what he has in mind is Western man and Christianity. Nor is he concerned with individualism in the dubious sense, but only that the individual, by a free personal surrender and willing acceptance of the consequences, should face the meaning of Christianity. Jung expects the Christian spirit to bring about a new change in man, a change which can be accomplished only by the individual changing *himself*, thus infusing new life into Christianity as a whole and not merely strengthening a particular creed or outward form. Hence Jung is saying nothing less than this: Christianity must become a personal experience—not merely a personal conviction as to the value of the generally accepted views, but an active ingredient in one's very life, something which one must acquire and bring to fruition for oneself, which cannot be taken over ready-made from others or recommended to others for their good. In this way Jung sets the individual in the very centre of religion as no Church has ever done.

Jung also opens up another channel of information for the clergyman, and that, astonishing though it may sound, is connected with *dogma*. What does dogma mean for many Protestant theologians today, and for many Catholic ones as well? Either they are convinced of its untruth, and they spend the greater part of their time convincing others of its untruth; or, for certain reasons, sometimes quite respectable reasons, they cling to the truth of the dogma and give themselves enormous pains trying to prove it. These pains can become positively convulsive when the theologian is, in his heart of hearts, something of a sceptic and yet refuses to admit it to himself. Then he preaches dogma at people and endeavours to convince them of its truth, generally with the result that those who should have ears to hear hear nothing, and no good is done at all. Jung, however, says that dogma can lay no claims to external truth and that it is extremely doubtful whether it can ever correspond to objective facts—indeed, in the case of many dogmas, it is obviously not so. But, on the other hand, the dogma is a *psychic reality*—that is, it contains certain psychic elements which are undoubtedly operative for the individual or mankind, and thus of the greatest significance.

For instance, it is pointless to ask whether the Virgin Birth is objectively true, but the primordial image of the Divine Child *behind* this dogma is most important psychologically, since it expresses the latent possibility of man's spiritual renewal by means of certain experiences.

Jung, therefore, urges the theologian to scrutinize dogma from this novel point of view. He would say that the theologian has to instil the ancient wisdom contained in the dogma into his sermons. This is a totally new attitude, and we should do well to take it very seriously. For we may be absolutely certain that a particular dogma would not have been invented had there not been cogent psychological reasons for it. Human beings created dogmas for certain definite reasons and purposes, and it is wrong to thrust them perfunctorily aside. On the other hand, it is most unsatisfactory, indeed quite pointless, when the sanctimonious preservation of traditional dogma merely leads to the limitation of human knowledge, as in the Catholic or orthodox Protestant use of dogma, or when constant appeals to dogma bring about a split between faith and religion on the one hand, and knowledge and science on the other, with the result that man's psychic unity is impaired. Certain branches of Protestantism are not entirely blameless in this respect. Jung tries to discover all he can about the psychological background of dogma and its aims, and his recognition that what is psychologically true has a psychological and therefore a human meaning—though it need not be objectively true—gives dogma a definite meaning and value of its own. The theologian will probably have to do a good deal of thinking on this new attitude to dogma; nevertheless, there is something tremendous in Jung's intimation that human experience and wisdom are laid down in dogma and symbol.

From this one can see what a far cry it is from classical psychoanalysis to Jung. Reik, a representative of psycho-analysis at its most anti-religious, wrote a book on *Das Dogma als Zwangsidee* (Dogma as a Compulsive Idea). The title alone is enough to show that he equates dogma with the pathological symptoms of psychic life, symptoms which, to the doctor, indicate neurosis. It was Freud himself who was responsible for this view, and Freud's labours with regard to religion can best be summed up by saying that he tried to cure mankind of religion. To his mind, religion was an illusion, by means of which psychically weak or unbalanced persons attempted to make the hard facts of reality endurable. There can be no doubt that such an abuse of religion exists. But this is to say nothing about the nature of true religion. Freud and his followers are of the opinion that, generally speaking, religion is being undermined by science. They regard psychoanalysis as an essential part of the new scientific enlightenment, and believe that, by laying bare the psychological motives, it will help people to rid themselves of illusion. Psychoanalysis wants to lead man to a sense of reality—as it understands reality—and free him and cure him altogether of religion, which it regards as, at bottom, superstition.

Jung adopts a totally different view. He approves religion as being an essential manifestation of psychic life. There is no question of his regarding it as a colossal aberration, a delusion, to be rejected on that account. At the same time he does not overlook the fact that all sorts of pathological phenomena can be detected in religion, and that a pathology of religious life would be very easy to compile. But he refuses to accept the idea that religion is in itself a symptom of psychic morbidity. On the contrary, he sees in the religious function one of the most important elements of the human psyche. That is why he tries, as a psychotherapist, to help all his patients along the road to the sort of religious experience they need. If Freud wants to cure people of religion, Jung wants to cure them through religion and give them a personal religion. The religious function is not the same for everybody—consequently, religion may mean very different things. To a quite extraordinary degree Jung is aware of the diversity of religious life, and tries to be as just as he can to every form of religion he meets. Those who read his writings attentively, however, will note after a time that he is rather on the side of a specific form of religion consisting in living processes which are, on the one hand, essential components of human experience, and, on the other, are happenings within some reality that transcends the individual—we could even say, happenings in God. Not that Jung ever goes so far as to say this: he would regard such an utterance as metaphysical, and metaphysics, in his view, is a pursuit which does not fit him as a psychologist. But if one reads Jung and, shall we say, Carus, together, one is sorely tempted to supplement Jung's thinking by Carus's metaphysical ideas. For the psychology of Jung, particularly his interpretation of unconscious processes in the collective psyche, would make an admirable foundation for a metaphysic in the sense intended by Carus, so admirable that it is well-nigh impossible to resist the temptation to take up the threads. Nor can one quite rid oneself of the suspicion that Jung himself is secretly of the same opinion.

Consider, for instance, Jung's view that God is first and foremost a psychological fact. He speaks of a God-image, by which he is not to be taken as saying that the individual has any power over this image. Although belonging to spiritual experience, the image and all such contents are "pathos" and themselves belong to those psychic powers which we may experience but with which we may not identify ourselves save at the cost of madness. In religious experience, therefore, certain processes are at work whose significance transcends personality. The individual becomes conscious of psychic contents which are of a supra-personal order. From this it is but a short step to the view that psychic reality is constantly realizing itself, or becoming conscious, in man, and that in man God is accomplishing his own transformation. The changes to which man is subject, his whole evolution, are in the last resort nothing less than a reflection of the Becoming of God—the pattern of emergent Deity. When Jung lays so much stress on religion's being born of the fullness of life, this has relevance here. We can also understand why Jung goes back to the doctrines of the relativity of God as formulated by the mystics. Such a view signifies that certain human occurrences have a meaning for God and that God in turn works on human life. Our human experience and suffering are thus related to what is going on in God.

We can say with some truth, then, that this places Jung in a spiritual current whose representatives in philosophy are generally reckoned among the so-called "life-philosophers." Carus, as a metaphysician, is one of them, likewise Schelling, Jakob Boehme, Max Scheler, and Ludwig Klages. Jung has affinities with this philosophical trend. So that it is not to be wondered at if mysticism figures in Jung's writings. And the above-mentioned thinkers, too, all refer to experiences known to the mystics: their theme is the changing and emerging God—a doctrine also to be met with in Rilke. This doctrine is closely connected with the doctrine of the relativity of God; indeed, it is its necessary counterpart. The changes in man reflect the events taking place in God, but the question is left open how far the connexion between God's life and man's is a causal one or whether we are here dealing with the simultaneous fulfilment of processes whose relations with our thoughts and intuitions cannot be explained, but only pointed out. Jung approaches these experiences as a psychologist only; they are not the basis of his "philosophy" as they were, explicitly or implicitly, for the thinkers we have mentioned.

Somewhere Jung has made the remark that he belongs to the extreme Left Wing in the Parliament of Protestantism. It would appear, therefore, that he reckons himself among the Protestants in the widest sense of the word. This classification of himself will not be admitted by many church-minded Protestants. It depends, of course, on what one means by Protestantism. Those who give most weight to the Church as a principle, or who stress fidelity to the letter of the ancient formulas and creeds, will hardly accept Jung as a champion of the Protestant spirit. But in a larger sense this appraisement of Jung's is quite right. He is one of those *outsiders* of Protestantism who sometimes give the orthodox more trouble, and cause them more displeasure, than all the other creeds and religions put together. Among these outsiders can be counted people like Herder and Hamann, Jakob Boehme, and—in more recent times— Franz Overbeck and Albert Schweitzer. They cannot be fitted into any denominational pattern, and yet they grow out of the Protestant spirit, not out of Catholicism. They express their views with unrelenting vigour and tartness, with no respect whatever for creed or Church politics. Sometimes they seem to be digging the grave for the whole corpus of orthodox thought. But as a rule, after the uproar about their heretical opinions and horror at their innovations have subsided, a good part of their thought seeps through into the general intellectual atmosphere, and even Protestantism summons up sufficient courage to digest much of what it initially rejected. Regarded from the viewpoint of the intellectual development of Protestantism, these outsiders generally signify the beginning of a new movement.

It is tempting, having placed Jung in this context, to compare him with Franz Overbeck. Overbeck, who was Professor of Church History in Basel, felt the conflict between theology and history at its deepest. In the end he could no longer reconcile theology with scientific principles, and declared that one has to choose between theology and science. One must make a clean break: either this or that. Either one is a theologian, and then one renounces science, or, if one wants to be a scientist, one must have no truck with theology. Overbeck chose the latter course. Jung is aware of a similar sharp cleavage: the cleavage between orthodox religion and personal religious experience. Membership of the Church gives you a religious creed, but if you belong to the Church you must renounce personal religious experience. Only if you break loose from the Church can you hope to come by the latter. So that here, too, the individual stands at the cross-roads, where a choice must be made, and a very fateful choice at that. Opting for the Church, you enter into a mighty religious inheritance; but this entails forgoing certain values necessary for the development of your own personality. If, on the other hand, you leave the Church, you must go the way of spiritual poverty, throwing away all means of defence against the perils of the soul—a renunciation which, for many people, is a hard lot indeed. Jung's views are further complicated by the fact that the Protestant Church is incapable of satisfying completely the psychic demands that a man makes of it, and that the Catholic Church alone fully realizes the church-principle. So that in Jung as in Overbeck we meet with a situation which demands far-reaching decisions from the individual, and both have much to say in criticism of the existing state of affairs.

With Jung, in contrast to Overbeck, criticism takes second place, since the main thing is his affirmative attitude and his unqualified desire to build up rather than to pull down. In this Jung finds himself far more in agreement with Albert Schweitzer, certainly the most caustic critic of orthodoxy that one can possibly imagine. Schweitzer's theological researches bid fair to demolish our whole interpretation of dogma as known so far, but then, by examining the content and meaning of early Christianity and by comparing it with other religions, he tries to bring out the essential value of Christianity. His object is to find some meaning in Christianity which will give people something to hold on to in life, a sense of direction in their work as well as in their ethical outlook.

Compared with Schweitzer, Jung has a totally different attitude to dogma. He is a psychologist, whereas the other is a theologian and historian. That is why Jung asks no questions about the objective truth or the ethical insight which may or may not be contained in dogma; all he looks for is the psychological facts expressed in it, asking what they mean for the person concerned. At the very outset, therefore, Jung is positive to the dogma, since he assumes that it must be taken as a psychological, not an objective, truth. As to whether, psychologically speaking, it "works," is something that is completely outside the range of scientific influence. Science can only establish whether it does or does not work in fact. But, in the last analysis, Jung comes to a conclusion regarding religion which is not so very unlike Schweitzer's. In Jung the overcoming of an inner conflict, the solution of the problem of opposites by a religious symbol or through religious experience, plays an important part. In Schweitzer, too, we come across this struggle to triumph over some contradiction or cleavage, namely that between ethics and knowledge. Ethics, or the will to morality, presupposes an affirmation of life, but knowledge of the world finds no grounds for this, no meaning which might serve as a durable foundation for any glorification of existence—on the contrary, knowledge spells negation. Hence, for Schweitzer, the thinking person is always faced with the decision between acceptance or rejection of life. These two things contradict one another dialectically, and there is no rational point of union between them. Schweitzer finds that a reconciliation is possible only in some ethical Christ-mythos which, being mystical, is irrational. Such is his solution of the problem of opposites.

In the matter of guilt as well, Jung and Schweitzer reach similar solutions. Jung expects the Protestant not to rid himself of guilt by confessing, but to take the experience of his guilt as an incentive to self-knowledge, and, by this means, to throw light on the background of his personality—in other words, the "shadow," as Jung calls it. In this way he will get the better of certain aspects of himself. Speaking of guilt, Schweitzer has remarked that a good conscience is an invention of the devil. Nevertheless, he does what he can to free the individual from the paralysing terrors of remorse, and to make him see that the experience of guilt can be a spur to ethical behaviour. Schweitzer's solution of the guilt-problem is a good example of what Jung calls the irrational reconciliation of opposites. Both men point clearly to the same sort of attitude.

If Schweitzer is the representative of a Christ-mysticism, we can find in Jung's attitude to religion an appeal to mystical experiences. In contrast to Schweitzer, he affirms not only Christ-mysticism but God-mysticism as well. So that though there may be differences between them which ought not to be overlooked or minimized, there are very considerable and significant areas of agreement. Their interests and respective fields of research lie far apart, yet both men are doctors ready to help all they can, not only their patients but, through their literary work, modern man himself. To him they seek to give counsel and guidance in that most central of all problems—religion. Their premises are different, their methods are different, but their answers to the pressing questions of the age have similarities which are not the result of coincidence; rather these have a common background and may thus provide material for very important discoveries concerning our situation, whether religious, psychological, or spiritual.

What Jung is seeking in regard to religion is the broadest and deepest possible understanding of religious life, and he wants to make religion, in whatever form it is practised, a living experience and a spiritual reality. He sees that modern man has reached a point where he no longer has anything to guide his life by and has, in consequence, lost all inner certainty. His questioning as to the meaning of existence has grown into a hard and temporarily insoluble problem. This state of intellectual and spiritual uncertainty is really a religious crisis. Jung tries to overcome it by a rediscovery of religion, which alone can convey vital experience. In some cases, Jung sees himself obliged to prepare the way for such experiences as will release a psychological change or, as we could fitly call it, a regeneration. In psychology he sees, further, a superlative instrument for understanding and interpreting all forms of religion, past and present. Thanks to the insight it gives us into our own personalities and psychic processes, it may, in Jung's view, finally produce a "constellation" of the psyche which will perhaps vouchsafe us altogether new religious experiences.

Psychology, however, is never merely the outcome of the desire for scientific knowledge; it rests on the deep-seated need to enlarge our consciousness and our conscious experience of the soul. Yet it should be noted that psychology can only prepare the way for these experiences and inner changes; it can never create the experiences and changes themselves. Whether these shall in fact occur and what they will bring us depends on psychic processes which we can, indeed, feel in ourselves, but about the nature and meaning of which we know absolutely nothing. We cannot compel them to happen, and we cannot influence or shape their contents in any way. We can only experience them passively.

The historical significance of Jung's work cannot be rightly assessed today. As Gebser so justly says, time alone will show whether this attempt on the part of science to get closer to the nature of religion will lead to an inner reconstruction or to a further undermining of it. However that may be, all those who are concerned with religion must take account of Jung's work. There is no point in retracing our steps behind him; we can only go forward along the trail he has blazed.

INDEX

Printed and bound by CPI Group (UK) Ltd, Croydon, CR0 4YY

01/11/2024

01782629-0004